Current Concepts and Controversies in Scaphoid Fracture Management

Editor

STEVEN L. MORAN

HAND CLINICS

www.hand.theclinics.com

Consulting Editor
KEVIN C. CHUNG

August 2019 • Volume 35 • Number 3

ELSEVIER

1600 John F. Kennedy Boulevard • Suite 1800 • Philadelphia, Pennsylvania, 19103-2899

http://www.theclinics.com

HAND CLINICS Volume 35, Number 3
August 2019 ISSN 0749-0712, ISBN-13: 978-0-323-68210-7

Editor: Lauren Boyle
Developmental Editor: Kristen Helm

Hand Clinics (ISSN 0749-0712) is published quarterly by Elsevier Inc., 360 Park Avenue South, New York, NY 10010-1710. Months of publication are February, May, August, and November. Business and Editorial Offices: 1600 John F. Kennedy Blvd., Ste. 1800, Philadelphia, PA 19103-2899. Customer Service Office: 3251 Riverport Lane, Maryland Heights, MO 63043. Periodicals postage paid at New York, NY and at additional mailing offices. Subscription price is $435.00 per year (domestic individuals), $813.00 per year (domestic institutions), $100.00 per year (domestic students/residents), $501.00 per year (Canadian individuals), $947.00 per year (Canadian institutions), $546.00 per year (international individuals), $947.00 per year (international institutions), and $256.00 per year (international and Canadian students/residents). Foreign air speed delivery is included in all *Clinics* subscription prices. All prices are subject to change without notice. **POSTMASTER:** Send address changes to *Hand Clinics*, Elsevier Health Sciences Division, Subscription Customer Service, 3251 Riverport Lane, Maryland Heights, MO 63043. Customer Service (orders, claims, online, change of address): Elsevier Health Sciences Division, Subscription **Customer Service, 3251 Riverport Lane, Maryland Heights, MO 63043. Tel: 1-800-654-2452 (U.S. and Canada); 314-447-8871 (outside U.S. and Canada). Fax: 314-447-8029. E-mail: journalscustomerservice-usa@elsevier.com (for print support); journalsonlinesupport-usa@elsevier.com (for online support)**.

Reprints. For copies of 100 or more of articles in this publication, please contact the Commercial Reprints Department, Elsevier Inc., 360 Park Avenue South, New York, New York 10010-1710. Tel.: 212-633-3874; Fax: 212-633-3820; E-mail: reprints@elsevier.com.

Hand Clinics is covered in *MEDLINE/PubMed (Index Medicus)*, *Current Contents/Clinical Medicine*, *EMBASE/Excerpta Medica*, and *ISI/BIOMED*.

Contributors

CONSULTING EDITOR

KEVIN C. CHUNG, MD, MS
Charles B.G. de Nancrede Professor of
Surgery, Professor of Plastic Surgery and
Orthopaedic Surgery, Chief of Hand Surgery,
Michigan Medicine, Assistant Dean for Faculty
Affairs, Associate Director of Global REACH,
University of Michigan Medical School, Ann
Arbor, Michigan, USA

EDITOR

STEVEN L. MORAN, MD
Professor of Plastic Surgery, Professor of
Orthopedic Surgery, Division of Plastic and
Reconstructive Surgery, Department of
Surgery, Mayo Clinic, Rochester, Minnesota,
USA

AUTHORS

PETER C. AMADIO, MD
Professor of Biomedical Engineering
and Orthopedics, College of Medicine,
Mayo Clinic, Rochester, Minnesota,
USA

KIMBERLY K. AMRAMI, MD
Professor of Radiology, Chair,
Division of Musculoskeletal Radiology,
Mayo Clinic, Rochester, Minnesota,
USA

CHELSEA C. BOE, MD
Resident Physician, Department of Orthopedic
Surgery, Mayo Clinic, Rochester, Minnesota,
USA

MICHELLE G. CARLSON, MD
Division of Hand and Upper Extremity Surgery,
Hospital for Special Surgery, New York, New
York, USA

ANDREA H.W. CHAN, MD, FRCSC
Assistant Professor, Toronto Western
Hospital Hand Program, University
Hospital Network, Toronto, Ontario,
Canada

KEVIN C. CHUNG, MD, MS
Charles B.G. de Nancrede Professor
of Surgery, Professor of Plastic Surgery
and Orthopaedic Surgery, Chief of Hand
Surgery, Michigan Medicine, Assistant
Dean for Faculty Affairs, Associate Director
of Global REACH, University of Michigan
Medical School, Ann Arbor, Michigan,
USA

BASSEM T. ELHASSAN, MD
Professor, Orthopedic Surgery, Mayo
Clinic, Rochester, Minnesota,
USA

KATE ELZINGA, MD
Clinical Lecturer, Section of Plastic Surgery, University of Calgary, Foothills Medical Centre, Calgary, Alberta, Canada

DIEGO L. FERNANDEZ, MD
Professor of Orthopedic Surgery, University of Bern, Bern, Switzerland

MATTHEW A. FRICK, MD
Assistant Professor of Radiology, Mayo Clinic, Rochester, Minnesota, USA

MIKE HAYTON, FRCS (Tr & Orth), FFSEM (UK)
Consultant Hand and Wrist Surgeon, Upper Limb Unit, Wrightington Hospital, Wigan, United Kingdom

JAMES P. HIGGINS, MD
Chief, Curtis National Hand Center, MedStar Union Memorial Hospital, Baltimore, Maryland, USA

PAK-CHEONG HO, MBBS, FRCS (Edinburg), FHKAM (Orthopaedic Surgery), FHKCOS
Chief of Service, Prince of Wales Hospital, Alice Ho Miu Ling Nethersole Hospital, Tai Po Hospital, Consultant, Division of Hand and Microsurgery, Department of Orthopaedics and Traumatology, Prince of Wales Hospital, Clinical Professor (Honorary), Faculty of Medicine, The Chinese University of Hong Kong, Hong Kong SAR

EDWARD W. JERNIGAN, MD
Division of Hand and Upper Extremity Surgery, Hospital for Special Surgery, New York, New York, USA

SANJEEV KAKAR, MD
Professor of Orthopedics, College of Medicine, Mayo Clinic, Rochester, Minnesota, USA

JANE M. MATSUMOTO, MD
Assistant Professor of Radiology, Mayo Clinic, Rochester, Minnesota, USA

STEVEN L. MORAN, MD
Professor of Plastic Surgery, Professor of Orthopedic Surgery, Division of Plastic and Reconstructive Surgery, Department of Surgery, Mayo Clinic, Rochester, Minnesota, USA

KYLE W. MORSE, MD
Division of Hand and Upper Extremity Surgery, Hospital for Special Surgery, New York, New York, USA

MOHAMED MORSY, MB, BCh
Division of Plastic Surgery, Rochester, Minnesota, USA; Department of Orthopedic Surgery, Assiut University Hospital, Assiut University, Assiut, Egypt

CHYE YEW NG, MBChB (Hons), FRCS (Tr & Orth), DipHandSurg (Br & Eur)
Consultant Hand and Peripheral Nerve Surgeon, Upper Limb Unit, Wrightington Hospital, Wigan, United Kingdom

MITCHELL A. PET, MD
Curtis National Hand Center, MedStar Union Memorial Hospital, Baltimore, Maryland, USA

SCHNEIDER K. RANCY, BA
Medical Student, College of Medicine, SUNY Downstate Medical Center, Brooklyn, New York, USA

PETER C. RHEE, DO, MS
Associate Professor, Department of Orthopedic Surgery, Mayo Clinic, Rochester, Minnesota, USA

M. DIYA SABBAGH, MBBS
Division of Plastic and Reconstructive Surgery, Department of Surgery, Mayo Clinic, Rochester, Minnesota, USA

GERNOT SCHMIDLE, MD
Attending, Priv-Doz, Department of Trauma Surgery, Medical University Innsbruck, Innsbruck, Austria

NICOLE M. SGROMOLO, MD
Orthopaedic Surgery Resident, Department of Orthopaedic Surgery, Brooke Army Medical Center, San Antonio, Texas, USA

NINA SUH, MD, FRCSC
Assistant Professor, Roth McFarlane
Hand and Upper Limb Centre, University
of Western Ontario, St. Joseph's
Hospital, London, Ontario,
Canada

SCOTT W. WOLFE, MD
Chief Emeritus, Hand and Upper
Extremity Service, Hospital for
Special Surgery, Professor of Orthopedic
Surgery, Weill Medical College of
Cornell University, New York, New York,
USA

**WING-YEE CLARA WONG, MBChB, MRCS,
FRCSEd (Orth), FHKAM (Orthopaedic
Surgery), FHKCOS**
Consultant, Hand Wrist Elbow and
Microsurgery Clinic, The Chinese University of
Hong Kong Medical Clinic, Clinical Associate
Professor (Honorary), Faculty of Medicine, The
Chinese University of Hong Kong, The Club
Lusitano, Central, Hong Kong SAR

**FEIRAN WU, MA, MB BChir (Cantab), FRCS
(Tr & Orth)**
Training Interface Group Fellow, Upper Limb
Unit, Wrightington Hospital, Wigan, United
Kingdom

Contents

The scaphoid is the most commonly fractured bone in the wrist but 20% to 40% of scaphoid fractures are radiographically occult. Delayed or misdiagnosis can have significant consequences with late complications such as nonunion, malunion, or the development of avascular necrosis in the proximal pole. After initial negative radiographs, advanced cross-sectional imaging, including CT and MRI, ultimately may provide more accurate and rapid diagnosis than conventional radiography. With chronic fractures, the preferred modality depends on the clinical question. New techniques are evolving that will further advance imaging for diagnosis and treatment of scaphoid fractures.

 Video content accompanies this article at http://www.hand.theclinics.com.

The scaphoid is the most commonly fractured carpal bone; despite its frequent injury, the diagnosis of fracture can be complicated by the presence of normal radiographs at the time of presentation. Clinical intuition can be increased by physical examination and immediately available modalities such as ultrasound within the emergency department. Definitive diagnosis should be made with computed tomography and magnetic resonance to verify the presence of displacement. This article provides an overview of the incidence and presentation of acute scaphoid fractures with a surgical focus on percutaneous dorsal screw fixation.

This article presents historical aspects, rationale, indications, planning, and execution of anterior interpositional bone grafting technique for unstable scaphoid nonunions. The author's original technique considers four points: (1) preoperative planning based on comparative anteroposterior radiographs in maximal ulnar deviation was used to calculate resection zone, size of the graft, and scaphoid length; (2) a volar approach was used; (3) an iliac crest wedge-shaped corticocancellous graft was interposed; and (4) Kirschner wires were inserted for fixation. Contemporary refinements of the technique including a modification to treat nonunions with failed previous screw fixation with tricks and hints and results are shown.

Internal fixation of the scaphoid using a plate has been reported in the literature as far back as 1977. Recently, a specific plate designed for scaphoids has been developed, which provides considerably more buttress support than intramedullary headless screws, and offers a reliable method of rigid internal fixation for complex fractures. Indications to use such a plate include complex acute fractures, such as those with significant waist comminution or steep reverse oblique fractures, and complex nonunions with central bone loss resulting from failed previous headless screw fixation. This is now the authors' preferred treatment for these injuries.

Scaphoid proximal pole fractures remain a surgical challenge because of high propensity for nonunion, osteonecrosis, and ultimately carpal collapse. Options for management of nonsalvageable proximal pole fractures include non-vascularized bone grafts, vascularized pedicled bone grafts, free vascularized bone flaps, and rib cartilage grafts. The proximal pole of the hamate can also serve as a replacement arthroplasty in the setting of proximal pole scaphoid nonunions with collapse, bone loss, and/or osteonecrosis. This novel graft addresses shortcomings of other graft choices by providing a local structural autograft solution with minimal donor site morbidity, correcting carpal collapse, reconstructing the scapholunate ligament, and mitigating the need for microvascular anastomosis.

 Video content accompanies this article at http://www.hand.theclinics.com.

Arthroscopic bone grafting (ABG) in difficult scaphoid delayed union and nonunion allows thorough assessment and comprehensive management for scaphoid fracture and its sequelae. It provides a favorable biological environment for bony healing and produces minimal trauma to the soft tissues, aiding in rehabilitation. With adequate training and experience, high union rates and satisfactory clinical outcomes can be achieved. Poor blood supply of the scaphoid is not a contraindication to bone grafting; union rates over 80% have been reported, comparable to other existing surgical methods. This article discusses the rationale, surgical techniques, and results of ABG.

Management of scaphoid nonunions requires thoughtful preoperative and intraoperative consideration to evaluate for scaphoid flexion or humpback deformity, carpal collapse, and proximal pole vascularity. Most scaphoid nonunions do not require vascularized bone grafts; however, in the setting of avascular necrosis of the proximal pole, vascularized bone grafts should be used to optimize union rates. In addition, scaphoid geometry and carpal stability must be restored to enhance functional outcomes.

Many hand surgeons argue that vascularized bone grafting is indicated in proximal pole avascular necrosis, prior failed surgery, or long-standing scaphoid nonunion.

However, the available evidence does not support improved treatment outcomes for vascularized bone grafting rather than traditional nonvascularized techniques. This article addresses the available evidence and examines the role of vascularized bone grafting in scaphoid nonunion treatment. It also identifies important factors that influence healing, clarifies the decision-making algorithm, and proposes areas for further research.

osteotomy and the use of structural graft to recreate anatomy and restore normal carpal motion. Clinical improvement of symptomatic scaphoid malunion can be reliably obtained with reconstruction, although the natural history and role for intervention in asymptomatic malunions remains unclear.

HAND CLINICS

SERIES OF RELATED INTEREST:

Clinics in Plastic Surgery
Orthopedic Clinics of North America
Physical Medicine and Rehabilitation Clinics of North America

THE CLINICS ARE AVAILABLE ONLINE!
Access your subscription at:
www.theclinics.com

Preface

Current Concepts and Controversies in Scaphoid Fracture Management

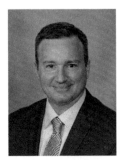

Steven L. Moran, MD
Editor

In 1980, my mentor, Dr William Cooney, wrote: "Historically, the scaphoid fracture has been subdivided into three types: the acute fracture, the delayed fracture, and the scaphoid nonunion. Controversy has developed with respect to the treatment of these fracture types."[1] Since 1980, the scaphoid has remained the most frequently fractured carpal bone, and yet its management is still a source of controversy. With almost four decades of study since Dr Cooney's article on a "rational approach" to scaphoid management, it is still difficult to say what is the gold standard for immobilization, the absolute indications for acute surgical repair, and the appropriate management of the nonunion. During my career as a surgeon, I have seen the clinical pendulum for the management of scaphoid nonunions swing from nonvascularized structural grafts, to pedicle vascularized grafts, to free flaps, to total arthroscopic repair. I still ask myself: "What is best for the patient?"

To help us try to answer many of the ongoing questions in the management of scaphoid fractures, we have called on some of the world's authorities to provide their perspective on current management. The text begins with new advancements in imaging of the scaphoid. We follow with an overview of the management of acute scaphoid fractures. We then focus on the more complex management issues surrounding scaphoid nonunions. Here, we cover the time-honored tips of master surgeon, Diego Fernandez, as well as newer techniques, including the use of volar plates, partial hamate autograft reconstruction, and pure arthroscopic management. In addition, we have asked for a new appraisal of the benefits of vascularized bone grafting: who needs a vascularized graft? Finally, we cover the complex issues of scaphoid management in the athlete and the healed malunion.

I would like to thank the authors for their outstanding articles as well as Kristen Helm and the team at Elsevier for their invaluable help in completing this issue of the *Hand Clinics*. We hope you learn something from reading it.

Steven L. Moran, MD
Division of Plastic Surgery
Mayo Clinic
200 First Street SW
Rochester, MN 55905, USA

E-mail address:
moran.steven@mayo.edu

REFERENCE

1. Cooney WP, Dobyns JH, Linscheid RL. Fractures of the scaphoid: a rational approach to management. Clin Orthop Relat Res 1980;149:90–7.

hand.theclinics.com

Imaging for Acute and Chronic Scaphoid Fractures

Kimberly K. Amrami, MD*, Matthew A. Frick, MD, Jane M. Matsumoto, MD

KEYWORDS

- MRI • Dynamic contrast enhancement • CT • Occult scaphoid fracture • 3-D modeling

KEY POINTS

- MRI is the optimal second test assessing a possible scaphoid fracture after a negative radiograph.
- Of scaphoid fractures, 20% to 40% are radiographically occult.
- When the fracture is visible on radiograph, computed tomography (CT) is the preferred test for further assessment of the fracture and for surgical planning.
- Cone beam CT and digital tomosynthesis have roles in determining progressive healing at a higher sensitivity than radiograph and at a lower cost than conventional CT.
- MRI with dynamic contrast enhancement may have a role is assessing the viability of bone before and after surgery but compelling data are lacking.

INTRODUCTION

The scaphoid is the most commonly fractured carpal bone and is most commonly fractured in active young adults. Scaphoid fractures are significant because of the potential complications such as nonunion, delayed union, or avascular necrosis (AVN), all of which are more likely in the setting of delayed diagnosis and treatment. Patients often present to the emergency department where non-hand specialists may see the patient, making the radiographic diagnosis even more critical. Unfortunately, up to 40% of acute scaphoid fractures are radiographically occult, even when radiographs are optimally performed and reviewed by a skilled interpreter[1] (**Fig. 1**). This presents a challenge to early diagnosis in the acute setting but the increasing availability of cross-sectional imaging, even in the emergency setting, presents an opportunity to reduce missed or delayed diagnoses.

ACUTE SCAPHOID FRACTURES

Radiography has traditionally been the starting point for imaging of the hand and wrist, especially in the setting of trauma. Initial imaging of the wrist should always include well-positioned posteroanterior (PA) and lateral views of the wrist.[2] Additional views, such as a pronated oblique and an ulnar deviated PA to fully extend the scaphoid, are often added to improve visualization. A retrospective study of 113 subjects with radiographically identified scaphoid fractures evaluated the types of views obtained and their impact on the diagnosis of the fracture. The investigators determined that fractures seen on specialized views, such as elongated or supinated oblique views, could be seen on other views, so that an appropriate radiograph imaging series in the case of suspected scaphoid fracture should include a PA, lateral, pronated oblique, and ulnar deviated PA.[3] It is rare but, occasionally, fractures of the proximal third of the scaphoid are best seen on the pronated oblique view (**Fig. 2**). Additional views, such as a supinated oblique or radially deviated PA, are of doubtful utility in the acute setting.

In addition to visualizing the fracture itself, it has long been suggested that secondary signs, such as the so-called scaphoid stripe sign, can be a useful adjunct to diagnosis.[4–6] In the normal and nontraumatic state there is lucent fat stripe at the

The authors have no financial or other conflicts to disclose.
Department of Radiology, Mayo Clinic, 200 1st Street Southwest, Rochester, MN 55905, USA
* Corresponding author.
E-mail address: amrami.kimberly@mayo.edu

hand.theclinics.com

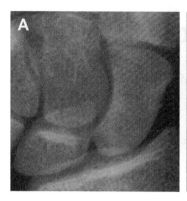
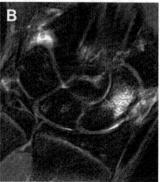

Fig. 1. Radiographically occult acute scaphoid fracture; imaging on the day of injury. (*A*) Photographically enlarged posteroanterior (PA) view of the wrist is negative. (*B*) Coronal T2-weighted MRI with fat suppression shows a fracture through the waist of the scaphoid with bone marrow edema.

radial aspect of the scaphoid on the PA view; the scaphoid stripe sign represents loss of the normal fat, which is replaced by soft tissue density, representing soft tissue edema or fluid (**Fig. 3**). A retrospective study of 78 confirmed scaphoid fractures showed that the stripe sign was present in 73 subjects; however, when compared with MRI, the sensitivity and specificity of the stripe sign is only 50%.[7] The stripe sign is present in about 30% of patients without a scaphoid fracture, making this a poor predictor of the presence of a radiographically occult fracture.[4,8,9]

Follow-up radiographs at 2 to 6 weeks has also been suggested as a strategy when scaphoid fracture is suspected, based on the theory that bone resorption at the fracture site will become more visible over time, confirming or excluding the presence of a fracture (**Fig. 4**). A study of radiographically occult scaphoid fractures confirmed by MRI looked at the sensitivity and specificity of follow-up radiographs from 10 to 50 days after the initial injury.[10] Of the 50 subjects included in this study, 35 had scaphoid fractures and 15 did not. Four expert observers (experienced orthopedic surgeons and radiologists) performed a blinded review with individual observer sensitivities ranging from 11% to 43%, with specificity in the 90th percentile; however, the negative predictive value was only 40%. Strikingly, interobserver reliability was poor at only 33%. Other studies have shown a kappa value of only 0.4 for radiographs obtained at the time of injury for the diagnosis of scaphoid fractures.[11] Considering that up to 36% of subjects suspected of having a scaphoid fracture actually have them, it is clear that, even with the high sensitivity of 70% to 90% reported in some studies,[12,13] radiography alone is inadequate to identify all acute scaphoid fractures. The consequences of both overtreatment and undertreatment are significant in terms of late complications, disability, and costs, making early and accurate diagnosis critical.[14] A recent study

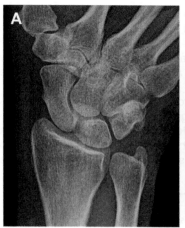
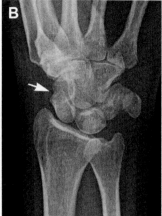
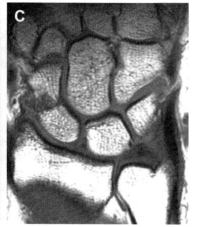

Fig. 2. (*A*) PA view of the wrist is negative. (*B*) Pronated oblique view of the wrist shows a scaphoid waist fracture with a positive scaphoid stripe sign (*arrow*) on the oblique image only. (*C*) Coronal T1-weighted MRI confirms the presence of a fracture.

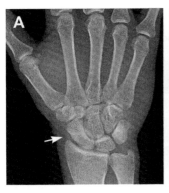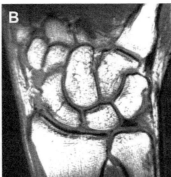

Fig. 3. (*A*) PA view of the wrist is negative for fracture. A positive scaphoid strip sign is present (*arrow*). (*B*) Coronal T1-weighted MRI shows the linear, nondisplaced fracture at the waist of the scaphoid.

proposed using MRI after a series of initial and follow-up radiographs at 7 days if there is a persistent concern for scaphoid fracture; however, this study noted significantly faster diagnosis with cross-sectional imaging, reducing the time to diagnosis from 24 to 9 days.[15] One finding of the study was the poor interobserver reliability for radiography (initial and follow-up) even among radiologists. Of note, in this study, 1 subject was immobilized for 67 days without a scaphoid fracture.

Other imaging options using radiographic techniques are of course available and have been proposed for the diagnosis of early scaphoid fractures. Polytomography, once a mainstay of hand and wrist imaging, has had something of a revival with the advent of digital tomosynthesis; however, data are lacking in terms of its value compared with cross-sectional imaging. A study of 35 subjects with clinically suspected scaphoid waist fractures and normal radiographs showed 3 fractures identified using tomosynthesis; however, 1 of these was also identified on conventional radiography, so that only 2 were only seen on the tomosynthesis studies.[16] As a further complication, this additional imaging test was performed 2 weeks after the initial trauma rather than at the time of injury, so that no real data are available about the utility of tomosynthesis in the acute setting. Digital tomosynthesis has not gained wide acceptance; both conventional and digital tomography have largely been replaced by computed tomography (CT).

CT is best used in the acute setting when the fracture is radiographically visible.[17] The high degree of resolution and multiplanar capability of CT makes it an ideal modality for surgical planning (**Fig. 5**). CT is highly sensitive to comminution, articular incongruity, and fracture fragment displacement, which can be critical in determining whether or not a so-called aggressive conservative approach to treatment can be used.[18] The overall sensitivity of conventional CT for acute scaphoid fractures has been reported to be similar to MRI but this depends to some degree on technique. Yin and colleagues[19] reported both higher sensitivity and almost perfect specificity (99.3%) with MRI. The choice of MRI or CT as a second test for radiographically occult scaphoid fractures largely depends on local availability in the acute setting.[14] However, when CT and MRI are both accessible, MRI is favored as a second test for the assessment of radiographically occult scaphoid fractures.[20] A recent European paper providing guidance for imaging scaphoid fractures according to evidence-based criteria recommends CT as the second test; however, the paper and guidelines do not distinguish between radiographically visible and radiographically occult fractures, and emphasizes assessment of the fracture pattern for surgical planning.[21]

A new technique using dual-energy CT (DECT) has been developed that shows promise for identifying acute scaphoid (and other) fractures. DECT uses 2 different levels of energy for the X-ray beam, which allows separation of some tissues based on their composition. It was originally used to separate urate from calcium oxalate stones in the kidneys and is currently used for assessing urate deposition in the hands and feet in patients with suspected gout.[22] A version of dual-energy technique allows calcium subtraction so that bone marrow edema becomes more apparent as increased density on the examination.[23] A small study of 3 subjects showed that the DECT technique with virtual calcium correlated with MRI, with 2 subjects having invisible or subtle fractures on radiograph and conventional radiograph, which were identified using the DECT technique when compared against MRI as a gold standard.[24] More study is needed but this technique is likely to have the best application in patient who cannot undergo an MRI either because of an implanted device incompatible with

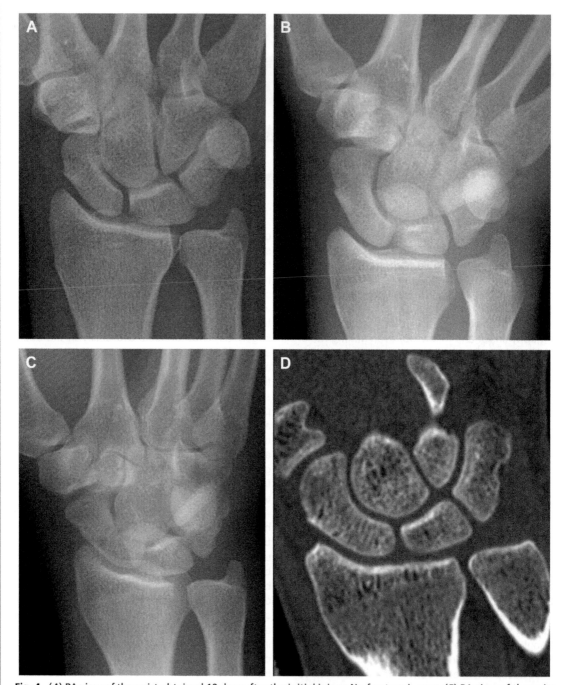

Fig. 4. (*A*) PA view of the wrist obtained 10 days after the initial injury. No fracture is seen. (*B*) PA view of the wrist obtained 2 weeks later does not show a fracture. PA view of the (*C*) wrist and (*D*) coronal CT obtained at 6 weeks from the time of injury show a nondisplaced, comminuted fracture of the distal scaphoid.

magnetic resonance, claustrophobia, or where MRI is not easily available after hours (**Fig. 6**).

Cone beam CT (CBCT) has undergone a revival recently, with dedicated systems available for the hand and wrist. CBCT was originally developed for use in dentistry but has been increasingly applied in other settings due to its low X-ray doses and the low cost of the equipment and siting compared with conventional CT. CBCT uses a conical X-ray source and 2-dimensional (2-D) flat detector to acquire images over an arc to reconstruct 2-D and 3-dimensional (3-D) imaging at

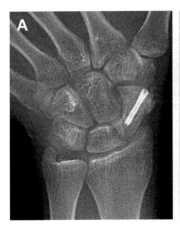
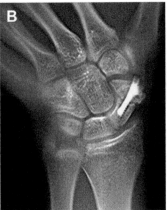

Fig. 5. (*A*) Coronal CT of the wrist showing screw fixation across a scaphoid fracture. (*B*) Coronal image from a digital tomosynthesis image of the same patient showing incomplete union of the scaphoid fracture. (*Courtesy of* GE Healthcare, Chicago, IL.)

relatively high resolution (**Fig. 7**). Although very limited in the evaluation of soft tissues and deeper osseous structures, CBCT has its most optimal application in the wrist. A hand-specific or wrist-specific unit approved by the US Food and Drug Administration is commercially available and can be installed in the space of a radiography room. The sensitivity of CBCT is reported as higher than radiographs for scaphoid fractures.[25,26] A single study by Borel and colleagues[25] comparing CBCT to MRI study showed 100% concordance between CBCT and MRI in subjects whose initial radiographs were negative for what the investigators describe as cortical fractures. CBCT is more susceptible to motion than conventional CT and beam-hardening artifacts can be more bothersome but, in most ways, CBCT for the wrist is as good as conventional CT for diagnostic purposes. The advantages are much lower siting costs, the ability to image patients sitting or standing up rather than lying prone with their arm in the superman position, and decreased ionizing radiation. These systems are commonly sited in outpatient facilities and are used for follow-up of healing

more often than for diagnosis in the acute setting; however, this may change as centers adopt this as an alternative to conventional CT.

Scintigraphy has traditionally been used as a second test for the assessment of radiographically occult scaphoid fractures but this is largely an artifact of the past.[27–29] Bone scan may be negative in the acute phase and it is rarely available after hours. Even when available, it is not ideal owing to its inability to distinguish fractures from bone contusions because both will the cause osteoclast or osteoblast activity, which is detected with conventional bone scans[30] (**Fig. 8**). Other types of nuclear medicine studies, such as single-photon emission CT, have been suggested due the ability to image at smaller fields of view with better resolution.[31] PET has been proposed for use with trauma but the cost, availability, and exposure to ionizing radiation make this an untenable option for diagnosis of fractures. Sonography has also been proposed for the diagnosis of acute scaphoid fractures. A recent meta-analysis of 7 studies of more than 10 subjects each investigating the performance of ultrasound (US) for the

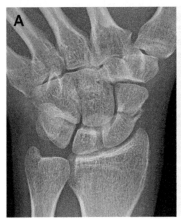
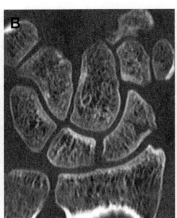
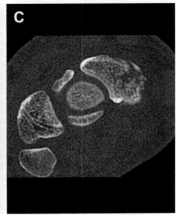

Fig. 6. Imaging obtained immediately after injury. (*A*) PA view of the wrist shows a fracture at the waist of the scaphoid. Coronal (*B*) and axial (*C*) images of the wrist show the fracture to be comminuted and distracted.

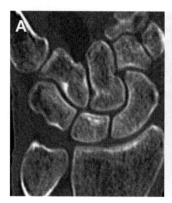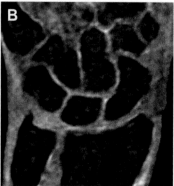

Fig. 7. DECT of the wrist obtained in a patient with a pacemaker unable to undergo MRI. (*A*) Conventional coronal CT image is negative for fracture. (*B*) Calcium-subtracted image showing no bone marrow edema present, confirming that no fracture is present. (*Courtesy of* K. Glazebrook, MD, Rochester, MN.)

diagnosis of scaphoid fractures included a total of 314 subjects.[32] The pooled estimate of the sensitivity of US for radiographically occult scaphoid fractures was 86% and the specificity was 83%. In this study, however, the reference standard was inconsistent between subjects and included CT, MRI, and even follow-up radiographs or clinical information. The investigators conclude that US can diagnose scaphoid fractures with a fairly high degree of accuracy and that the use of US is more cost-effective than empiric immobilization when CT and MRI are not available. The relevance of these findings is uncertain because musculoskeletal US is complex to perform and highly operator-dependent. The other significant limitation of US is its inability to identify other carpal and wrist fractures, which can be seen when patients present with snuffbox tenderness, which can be present in up to 20% of cases in which scaphoid fracture is suspected.[33] At this time, US cannot be considered a reliable second

imaging test for detecting scaphoid fractures at most centers.

MRI remains the gold standard for the diagnosis of radiographically occult scaphoid fractures.[20,34] Sensitivity has been reported in the 95% to 100% range and specificity is consistently at or near 100%. T2-weighted MRI with fat suppression is exquisitely sensitive to bone marrow edema; if bone marrow edema is absent, there is no fracture. This is the 1 instance in MRI in which lower field strength or a dedicated extremity MRI with lower image quality is not a limitation. Interobserver reliability is nearly perfect (kappa values reported as high as 0.953), making fracture detection less dependent on reader experience than almost any other test in radiology. Optimal pulse sequences for fracture detection include a fluid-sensitive sequence with fat suppression, such as T2-weighted fast spin-echo with fat suppression or short tau inversion recovery (STIR) to visualize the edema. A T2*-weighted gradient-echo

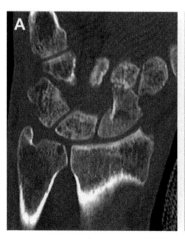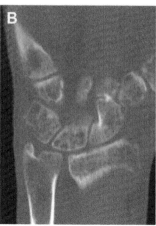

Fig. 8. (*A*) Conventional coronal CT image showing an ununited fracture with resorption at the scaphoid waist. (*B*) Same patient was imaged 4 weeks later using CBCT with coronal reconstruction.

sequence shows lower sensitivity (14% compared with 100% for STIR) and should not be used for this purpose. Diagnostic accuracy can be improved by the addition of a high-resolution T1-weighted series to visualize a fracture line. This can be important to make the distinction between a true fracture and a bone contusion (**Fig. 9**). A limited study including only coronal T1 and fluid-sensitive T2 with fat suppression is usually more than adequate to make the diagnosis.

MRI also has increased accuracy for identifying other pathologic conditions that may present with symptoms similar to a scaphoid fracture, such as snuffbox tenderness, or in association with a scaphoid fracture (**Fig. 10**). In a series of 195 subjects who underwent MRI for a clinically suspected scaphoid fracture and negative radiographs, 51% were normal, 19% had scaphoid fractures, and 17.4% had other fractures of either the carpal bones or distal radius.[33] This was a prospective study; almost 40% of subjects had a fracture of some kind and MRI changed management in 92% of cases. MRI has been evaluated for fracture displacement and alignment for surgical planning but, in general, CT is preferred due to its multiplanar capability and inherently higher spatial resolution.[18]

The cost of MRI is sometimes cited as problematic for its use in detecting occult scaphoid fractures but this fails to take into consideration costs related to follow-up examinations, unnecessary immobilization, and subsequent loss of productivity. Yin and colleagues[35] found that there were reduced costs with the use of immediate cross-sectional imaging to diagnose radiographically occult scaphoid fractures; however, other analyses, both retrospective and prospective, have

shown mixed results. Many of these studies have been performed in countries with nationalized healthcare, which is complicated to compare to a fee-for-service system such as the United States.[36] Study design has varied considerably between these studies in terms of timing of MRI relative to the injury, which also limits comparisons but, in general, when all factors are considered there is a societal cost savings to early use of advanced imaging for radiographically occult scaphoid fractures.[37] One recent decision analysis model performed in the United States comparing empiric casting, CT, and MRI, showed a significant advantage in both cost and morbidity with the use of immediate of advanced imaging, with the highest sensitivity for MRI and high specificity for CT.[14] Rua and colleagues[38] have proposed a randomized, prospective trial (SMaRT) to assess the utility of MRI against 4-view radiography by determining primary and secondary outcomes and costs of the total episode of care in the United Kingdom. Although perhaps not completely generalizable, this should yield important information about the total cost of care and impact on clinical outcomes when MRI is used as a primary diagnostic tool for wrist fractures.

CHRONIC SCAPHOID FRACTURES

CT is commonly used after the initial diagnosis, either by radiograph or MRI, to determine the degree of comminution and any displacement of fracture fragments[39] (**Fig. 11**). Imaging of scaphoid fractures after the initial diagnosis and treatment is primarily driven by the need for evaluation of healing and for the assessment of potential

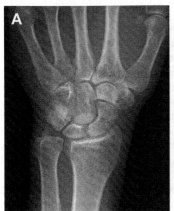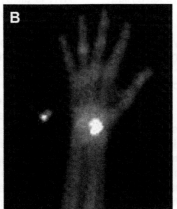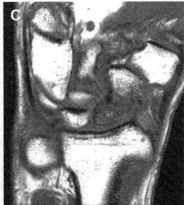

Fig. 9. (A) PA view of the wrist showing a minimally displaced fracture of the scaphoid, which was initially read as negative for fracture. (B) Delayed phase image from a 3-phase bone scan shows avid update in the region of the scaphoid. (C) Coronal T1-weighted MRI confirms the presence of a fracture in the scaphoid and excludes other carpal fractures.

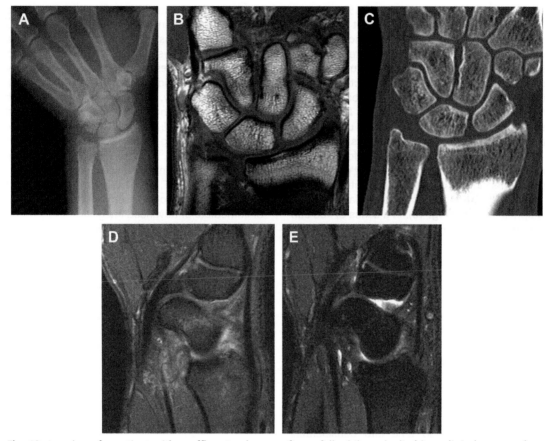

Fig. 10. Imaging of a patient with snuffbox tenderness after a fall while rock climbing; clinical concern for a scaphoid fracture was high. (*A*) Ulnar deviated PA view of the wrist is negative for fracture. (*B*) Coronal T1-weighted MRI of the wrist is negative for fracture. (*C*) Coronal CT image is also negative for fracture. (*D*) Sagittal T2-weighted MRI with fat suppression obtained at the time of image *B* shows an indistinct linear area of bone marrow edema at the scaphoid waist. In the absence of a low signal line on T1, this is consistent with a contusion rather than a fracture. (*E*) Sagittal T2-weighted MRI with fat suppression obtained 6 weeks later after cast immobilization shows complete resolution of the bone marrow edema seen in image *D*.

complications or associated findings, such as ligamentous injury, sustained with the original trauma.[40]

Primary union can be assessed by radiography in some cases but CT (either conventional or CBCT) is the optimal modality for determining trabecular bridging.[41,42] Partial or complete healing can be judged by serial imaging and patients can be imaged with a cast in place. If a screw or other fixation has been placed, this may cause some artifact but, in general, the hollow, percutaneous titanium screws used for fixating scaphoid fractures create less artifact for both MRI and CT than other types of metal or devices[43] (**Fig. 12**). Carpal alignment is better judged with radiography due to the positioning required for CT, which generally involves having the wrist supinated against some degree of at least passive resistance.

AVN is always a concern after scaphoid fractures, especially those involving the proximal third of the bone. CT in the early phases of healing can be misleading because increased density may be seen in the proximal fragment due to bone marrow edema and healing rather than to the development of AVN.[44] Care must be taken to not overdiagnose AVN in the first few months after treatment. If bone grafting has been performed, CT is the preferred modality for assessing incorporation of the graft at the fracture site but it cannot assess the viability of the graft (**Fig. 13**). For the assessment of graft viability and to exclude the presence of AVN, MRI is the preferred but not perfect modality. As with CT, MRI can be performed with a cast in place or in a patient who has undergone fixation and/or bone grafting as treatment; however, image quality with MRI is usually degraded by the presence of metal despite the use of metal suppression

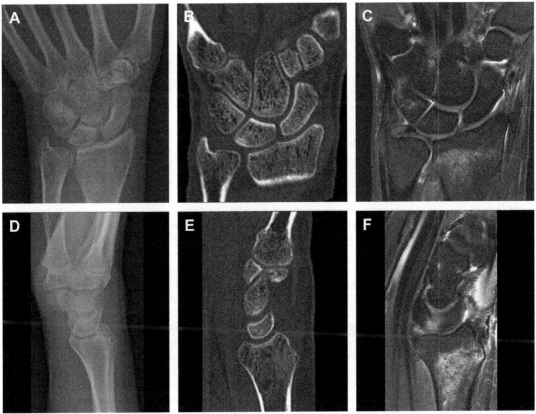

Fig. 11. Patient presented to the emergency department after a fall on an outstretched hand with high suspicion for a scaphoid fracture on physical examination. (*A*) PA and (*D*) lateral radiograph, (*B*) coronal and (*E*) sagittal CT images, and (*C*) coronal and (*F*) sagittal T2-weighted MRIs of the wrist show a nondisplaced fracture of the distal radius, which was missed on both radiograph and CT at the time of presentation. No scaphoid or other carpal fracture is present.

techniques to mitigate the susceptibility artifacts often seen. Contrast-enhanced DECT has been used experimentally to assess scaphoid proximal pole vascularity in a group of high-risk subjects in a small study but the results cannot be broadly applied without additional study.[45]

CT has significant value for assessing deformity that may indicate a malunion, especially when 3-D imaging can be performed and the carpal bones virtually disarticulated.[46–48] This can be done unilaterally but is best when the noninjured wrist can be imaged to determine asymmetry and plan

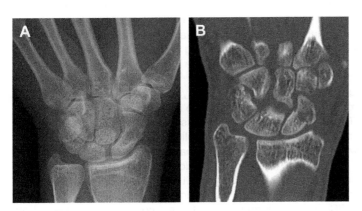

Fig. 12. (*A*) PA of the wrist showing a scaphoid waist fracture with resorption at the fracture site. (*B*) Coronal CT image of the wrist shows the resorption as well as 1 to 2 mm of displacement not appreciated on radiograph.

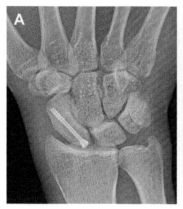 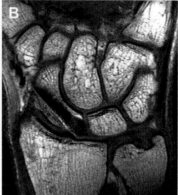 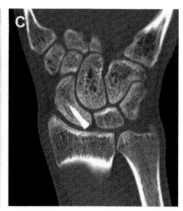

Fig. 13. (*A*) PA view of the right wrist shows screw fixation across a healed scaphoid waist fracture. (*B*) Coronal T1-weighted MRI confirms healing but there is some mild artifact associated with the screw. (*C*) Coronal CT image confirms complete healing and shows the proximal screw head located within the radiocarpal joint.

for surgery to restore normal morphology and function.[49] This necessarily involves additional radiation exposure but the effect of the small amount of radiation to an extremity with modern low-dose CT is not significant in a skeletally mature adolescent or adult. Caution should be exercised about the relative risk and benefit when imaging children.

A healing scaphoid fracture on MRI will generally show progressive obliteration of the fracture line and cortical and trabecular bridging can often be assessed on T1-weighted images; however, CT and even tomosynthesis are more sensitive than MRI for actual fracture healing.[50] There is commonly bone marrow edema on MRI, which can be present in the scaphoid for an extended period of time and which may or may not correlate with symptoms such as pain. MRI may also be helpful in assessing possible ligamentous injury, which may not have been appreciated or addressed at the time of the initial injury; for example, contusions of the scapholunate ligament are common but tears may also be seen, consistent with the common mechanism of injury of falling on an outstretched hand. Dynamic contrast enhancement has been proposed to assess healing of scaphoid fractures with MRI but, in general, this would be reserved for instances of delayed or nonunion or suspected AVN.[51]

Determining whether or not AVN is present on MRI is more complicated. The healing phase as noted is associated with bone marrow edema but this can also be seen in early AVN. The preservation of marrow fat on T1-weighted imaging has been thought to be a sign of preserved vascularity.[52] A recent study showed this to be an acceptable predictor but with accuracy only at 79% with a small sample of 18 subjects.[53] In this study, fluid-sensitive sequences (ie, STIR) were

deemed to be nonspecific and other studies have shown that bone marrow edema is present in 80% to 90% of viable and nonviable scaphoids, respectively.[54] In the presence of metal, even making these limited observations can be difficult.

MRI with dynamic contrast enhancement has been suggested as a tool for determining whether or not the proximal post of the scaphoid is viable after fracture (**Fig. 14**). Dynamic enhancement produces a curve of enhancement that can be done for both the scaphoid and a normal carpal bone as a control. Image subtractions can also be performed to visually assess the degree of enhancement in the carpal bones (**Fig. 15**). There is controversy regarding the timing of dynamic enhancement or whether or not delayed enhancement on its own can make the distinction between AVN and viable bone.[55] Published studies are contradictory,[54,56,57] with some indicating that the curve obtained with dynamic enhancement correlates better with surgical grading of vascularity and others saying that there is no added value for dynamic enhancement with time intensity curves. Most studies show that contrast-enhanced MRI is better than noncontrast MRI for assessing scaphoid vascularity but even that is hard to truly determine owing to the small numbers of subjects included and the lack of technical consistency between studies.[55,58] There have been studies suggesting that dynamic contrast-enhanced MRI may have a role in patient selection for vascularized bone grafts of the scaphoid.[53,59] Perhaps the best application for dynamic contrast enhancement may be for assessing vascularized bone grafts.[60] Normalization of the enhancement of the bone graft compared with the surrounding bone is a good indicator of intact vascularity. Unfortunately, it is common to see both

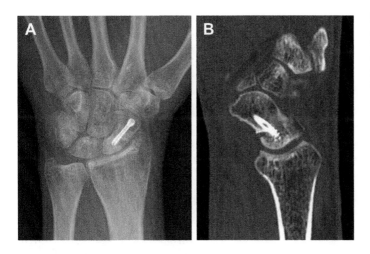

Fig. 14. (*A*) PA view of the wrist showing screw fixation across the scaphoid with a vascularized bone graft. Note donor site in the distal radius. (*B*) Sagittal CT image shows complete incorporation of the graft.

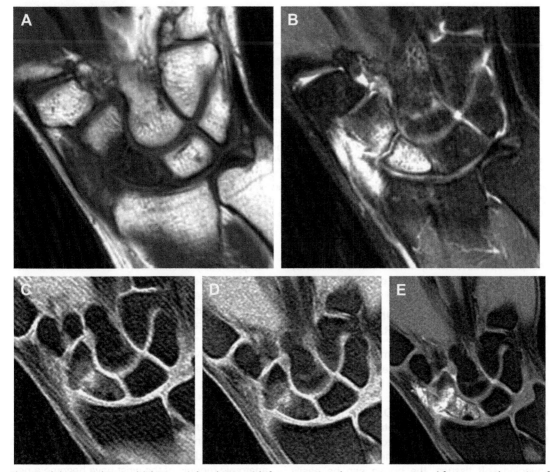

Fig. 15. (*A*) Coronal T1 and (*B*) T2-weighted MRI with fat saturation showing an ununited fracture at the waist of the scaphoid. There is very low T1 signal in the proximal portion of the scaphoid. Bone marrow edema is present on the (*B*) fluid-sensitive image. T1-weighted spoiled gradient-recalled (SPGR) images with fat suppression obtained at (*C*) 30 seconds, (*D*) 60 seconds, and (*E*) 2 minutes after the administration of intravenous contrast. Enhancement in the proximal pole indicates intact vascularity, which was later shown at surgery.

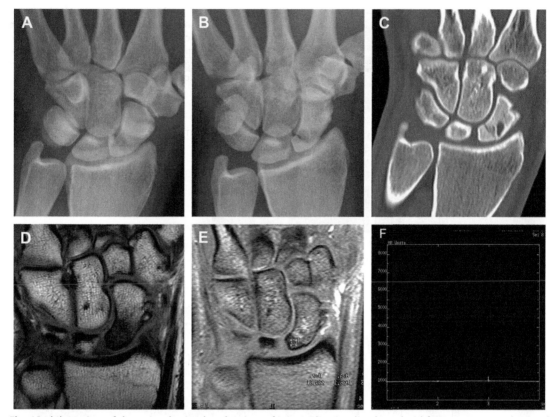

Fig. 16. (*A*) PA view of the wrist obtained at the time of injury. The visualized scaphoid fracture was not detected at that time. (*B*) PA view of the wrist obtained 3 months later showing the ununited fracture of the proximal pole of the scaphoid with increased density in the proximal pole fragment. (*C*) Coronal CT of the wrist at the time of image *B* showing the ununited fracture and marked increased density in the proximal pole, worrisome for AVN. (*D*) Coronal T1-weighted MRI showing very low signal in the proximal pole fragment, worrisome for AVN. (*E*) Image from dynamic enhancement series showing no enhancement in the proximal pole fragment, where a region of interest has been marked. (*F*) Time-intensity curve of contrast uptake in the proximal pole fragment is completely flat, consistent with AVN, which was proven at surgery.

percutaneous screws and other types of metal in the postoperative wrist, which can significantly limit the value of MRI for these patients.

THREE-DIMENSIONAL IMAGING AND MODELING OF SCAPHOID FRACTURES

3-D modeling of bone has dramatically improved with the advent of isotropic or near isotropic imaging techniques for both CT and MRI. Although CT acquisitions are not volumetric, thin sections with overlap will allow seamless 3-D virtual models to be created, which can be rotated and viewed from different perspectives. Because of the large density difference between the bone and surrounding soft tissues, the bones can be easily segmented and isolated. Blood vessels and tendons can also be layered into the images, depending on the techniques of acquisition. The carpal bones can be disarticulated to visualize the

individual surfaces and morphology of each bone. As previously mentioned, the contralateral side can be imaged for comparison, and to facilitate morphologic and functional reconstructions.[49,61]

3-D imaging with MRI is more complicated due to the time required and to limitations in tissue contrast and resolution with available techniques. MRI can provide additional value with differentiating soft tissues but segmentation is more difficult.[62,63] The creation of 3-D models, both virtual and concrete, can be used for surgical planning, as well as for patient education.[64]

High-resolution CT imaging has merged with rapidly evolving 3-D printing technology to allow a new way of displaying wrist imaging. 3-D printed anatomic models of the wrist have become a new useful tool for surgical care. 3-D printing technology developed in the 1980s as a method of creating inexpensive prototypes for manufacturing. It merged with medical imaging technology beginning

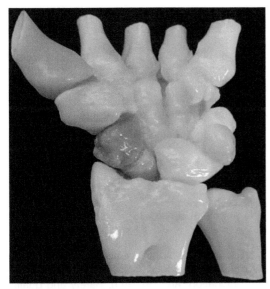

Fig. 17. Life-sized 3-D printed model of a wrist in a patient with a chronically ununited scaphoid fracture (distal pole of the scaphoid is gray).

in the 1990s for use in oral maxillary facial surgery. In the past decade, 3-D printing from imaging data has extended to other areas of medicine, most notably orthopedic, cardiac, and plastic surgery.

3-D printing of wrist anatomic models has begun to be used as aids in planning surgery. Common indications for 3-D printed models include wrists of patients with chronic deformities from scaphoid and lunate fractures, and congenital or acquired deformities of the distal radial ulnar joint (**Fig. 16**). Creation of the models is relatively straightforward. An important first step is image data acquisition. High-resolution imaging data with thin slices and soft kernel in a single acquisition covering the area of interest is obtained. The DICOM imaging data are transferred into dedicated software in which the bones of interest are segmented or separated from the adjacent anatomy on each image. The segmented bones are converted into a virtual 3-D image and then processed using computer-aided diagnosis (CAD) software into a 3-D printing–compatible file. These files are a surface mesh composed of triangles. The files are exported to a 3-D printer with a software program that takes the additional step of slicing the files into horizontal layers. The 3-D printer directs the printer to lay down thin layers of material in a sequential additive fashion according to the slicing design. These layers accumulate to create an anatomic model, which is a life-size 3-D physical display of the imaging data (**Fig. 17**).[65]

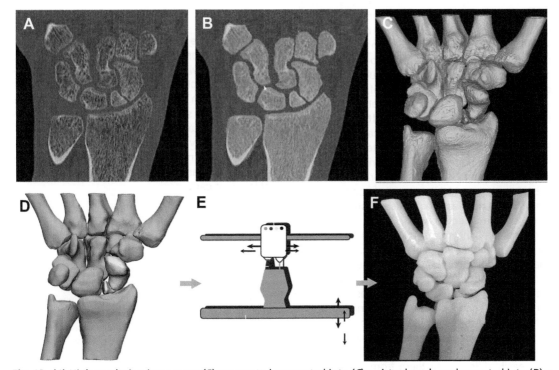

Fig. 18. (A) High-resolution images are (B) segmented, converted into (C) a virtual mask, and exported into (D) a stereolithography file for (E) 3-D printing, to produce (F) an anatomic physical model.

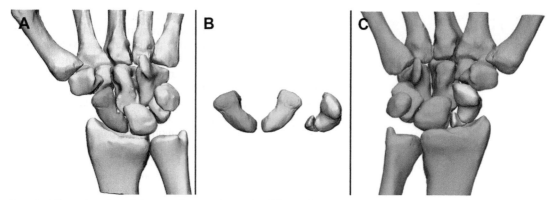

Fig. 19. Mirror imaging. (*A*) Normal, opposite wrist. (*B*) Scaphoid models showing the normal side, mirrored abnormal side, and original abnormal model with fracture. (*C*) Wrist with abnormal scaphoid.

There are many types of 3-D printers with a wide range of costs available and new ones are actively being developed. The printers have varying speed of printing, layer thickness, material type, colors, support material, and postprocessing requirements depending on the type of printing technology used. There are, although limited, sterilizable and biocompatible materials available.

The 3-D printed wrist model can be a life-sized physical representation of the individual patient's wrist bones using their own CT imaging data. The whole wrist or any desired separate subset of wrist bones can be printed. The bones can be magnified to any desired size and a scaled-up version printed. These physical models offer additional multisensory comprehension compared with 2-D imaging because they can be touched, rotated, and turned in any direction. The models help the surgeon to more fully understand the bony anatomy and relationships of the wrist. The increased comprehension of critical anatomy contributes to surgical planning (**Fig. 18**).

A unique feature of virtual surgical planning and 3-D printing is the ability to create mirror-image models of the normal opposite wrist to compare with the abnormal wrist. The mirror-image normal wrist serves to highlight and accentuate the abnormal boney features and anatomic relationships of the affected wrist. Both the affected abnormal and the mirror-image model can also be used in virtual surgical planning. The mirror-image model can be superimposed on the abnormal side to aid in planning the optimal osteotomy to the affected bone. These proposed surgical cuts can be simulated using computer software and the resulting cut bones can then be printed and used as surgical aids. Mirror-image models are often printed in a separate color to help easily differentiate them from the abnormal side (**Fig. 19**).[61]

3-D printing of imaging data is a rapidly evolving field in medicine and is being used in clinical practice, education, and research. Safety and quality assurance standards for 3-D printing from medical imaging data are developing with quality control programs for evaluation of accuracy.[66] Models are imprinted with a unique patient identifier, sidedness, and whether they are mirror imaged. Medical centers are establishing operations for model ordering and documentation. Reimbursement with establishment of current procedural terminology codes through the American Medical Association is being pursued.

SUMMARY

Imaging can be a powerful tool in the diagnosis of acute and chronic injury to the scaphoid. Surgical planning, follow-up, and assessment of late complications, such as AVN, delayed union, and nonunion, can be performed with techniques tailored for the specific indication. Although all imaging of the hand and wrist begins with radiography, high-value cross-sectional imaging, including 3-D modeling, can contribute to cost-effectiveness and improved outcomes in the total episode of care.

REFERENCES

1. Cooney WP 3rd. Scaphoid fractures: current treatments and techniques. Instr Course Lect 2003;52: 197–208.
2. Amrami KK, Berger RA. Radiology corner: review of plain radiographs. J Am Soc Surg Hand 2005;5(1): 4–7.
3. Cheung GC, Lever CJ, Morris AD. X-ray diagnosis of acute scaphoid fractures. J Hand Surg Br 2006; 31(1):104–9.
4. Annamalai G, Raby N. Scaphoid and pronator fat stripes are unreliable soft tissue signs in the

detection of radiographically occult fractures [see comment]. Clin Radiol 2003;58(10):798–800.

5. Dias JJ, Finlay DB, Brenkel IJ, et al. Radiographic assessment of soft tissue signs in clinically suspected scaphoid fractures: the incidence of false negative and false positive results. J Orthop Trauma 1987;1(3):205–8.

6. Terry DW Jr, Ramin JE. The navicular fat stripe: a useful roentgen feature for evaluating wrist trauma. Am J Roentgenol Radium Ther Nucl Med 1975; 124(1):25–8.

7. Cetti R, Christensen SE. The diagnostic value of displacement of the fat stripe in fracture of the scaphoid bone. Hand 1982;14(1):75–9.

8. Dobyns JH, Linscheid RL. Fractures and dislocations of the wrist. In: Rockwood CA, Green DP, editors. Fractures in adults, vol. 1, 2nd edition. Philadelphia: JB Lippincott; 1984. p. 411–23.

9. Schmitt R, Rosenthal H, Deutsche Gesellschaft fur U. Imaging of scaphoid fractures according to the new S3 guidelines. Rofo 2016;188(5):459–69.

10. Low G, Raby N. Can follow-up radiography for acute scaphoid fracture still be considered a valid investigation? Clin Radiol 2005;60(10):1106–10.

11. Tiel-van Buul MM, van Beek EJ, Broekhuizen AH, et al. Radiography and scintigraphy of suspected scaphoid fracture. A long-term study in 160 patients [see comment]. J Bone Joint Surg Br 1993;75(1): 61–5.

12. Brondum V, Larsen CF, Skov O. Fracture of the carpal scaphoid: frequency and distribution in a well-defined population. Eur J Radiol 1992;15(2):118–22.

13. Leslie IJ, Dickson RA. The fractured carpal scaphoid. Natural history and factors influencing outcome. J Bone Joint Surg Br 1981;63-B(2): 225–30.

14. Karl JW, Swart E, Strauch RJ. Diagnosis of occult scaphoid fractures: a cost-effectiveness analysis. J Bone Joint Surg Am 2015;97(22):1860–8.

15. Wijetunga AR, Tsang VH, Giuffre B. The utility of cross-sectional imaging in the management of suspected scaphoid fractures. J Med Radiat Sci 2019; 66(1):30–7.

16. Geijer M, Borjesson AM, Gothlin JH. Clinical utility of tomosynthesis in suspected scaphoid fracture. A pilot study. Skeletal Radiol 2011;40(7):863–7.

17. Krimmer H. Management of acute fractures and nonunions of the proximal pole of the scaphoid. J Hand Surg Br 2002;27(3):245–8.

18. Bhat M, McCarthy M, Davis TR, et al. MRI and plain radiography in the assessment of displaced fractures of the waist of the carpal scaphoid. J Bone Joint Surg Br 2004;86(5):705–13.

19. Yin ZG, Zhang JB, Kan SL, et al. Diagnosing suspected scaphoid fractures: a systematic review and meta-analysis. Clin Orthop Relat Res 2010; 468(3):723–34.

20. Amrami KK. Radiology corner: diagnosing radiographically occult scaphoid fractures - What's the best second test? J Am Soc Surg Hand 2005;5(3): 134–8.

21. Schmitt R, Heinze A, Fellner F, et al. Imaging and staging of avascular osteonecroses at the wrist and hand. Eur J Radiol 1997;25(2):92–103.

22. Lee SK, Jung JY, Jee WH, et al. Combining non-contrast and dual-energy CT improves diagnosis of early gout. Eur Radiol 2019;29(3):1267–75.

23. Pache G, Krauss B, Strohm P, et al. Dual-energy CT virtual noncalcium technique: detecting posttraumatic bone marrow lesions–feasibility study. Radiology 2010;256(2):617–24.

24. Dareez NM, Dahlslett KH, Engesland E, et al. Scaphoid fracture: bone marrow edema detected with dual-energy CT virtual non-calcium images and confirmed with MRI. Skeletal Radiol 2017; 46(12):1753–6.

25. Borel C, Larbi A, Delclaux S, et al. Diagnostic value of cone beam computed tomography (CBCT) in occult scaphoid and wrist fractures. Eur J Radiol 2017;97:59–64.

26. Neubauer J, Benndorf M, Ehritt-Braun C, et al. Comparison of the diagnostic accuracy of cone beam computed tomography and radiography for scaphoid fractures. Sci Rep 2018;8(1):3906.

27. Brismar J. Skeletal scintigraphy of the wrist in suggested scaphoid fracture. Acta Radiol 1988;29(1): 101–7.

28. Fowler C, Sullivan B, Williams LA, et al. A comparison of bone scintigraphy and MRI in the early diagnosis of the occult scaphoid waist fracture. Skeletal Radiol 1998;27(12):683–7.

29. Bellmore MC, Cummine JL, Crocker EF, et al. The role of bone scans in the assessment of prognosis of scaphoid fractures. Aust N Z J Surg 1983;53(2): 133–7.

30. Karantanas A, Dailiana Z, Malizos K. The role of MR imaging in scaphoid disorders. Eur Radiol 2007; 17(11):2860–71.

31. Querellou S, Arnaud L, Williams T, et al. Role of SPECT/CT compared with MRI in the diagnosis and management of patients with wrist trauma occult fractures. Clin Nucl Med 2014;39(1):8–13.

32. Kwee RM, Kwee TC. Ultrasound for diagnosing radiographically occult scaphoid fracture. Skeletal Radiol 2018;47(9):1205–12.

33. Brydie A, Raby N. Early MRI in the management of clinical scaphoid fracture. Br J Radiol 2003; 76(905):296–300.

34. Murthy NS. The role of magnetic resonance imaging in scaphoid fractures. J Hand Surg Am 2013;38(10): 2047–54.

35. Yin ZG, Zhang JB, Gong KT. Cost-effectiveness of diagnostic strategies for suspected scaphoid fractures. J Orthop Trauma 2015;29(8):e245–52.

36. Saxena P, McDonald R, Gull S, et al. Diagnostic scanning for suspected scaphoid fractures: an economic evaluation based on cost-minimisation models. Injury 2003;34(7):503–11.

37. Rua T, Parkin D, Goh V, et al. The economic evidence for advanced imaging in the diagnosis of suspected scaphoid fractures: systematic review of evidence. J Hand Surg Eur Vol 2018;43(6):642–51.

38. Rua T, Vijayanathan S, Parkin D, et al. Rationale and design of the SMaRT trial: a randomised, prospective, parallel, non-blinded, one-centre trial to evaluate the use of magnetic resonance imaging in acute setting in patients presenting with suspected scaphoid fracture. Clin Trials 2018;15(2):120–9.

39. Gilley E, Puri SK, Hearns KA, et al. Importance of computed tomography in determining displacement in scaphoid fractures. J Wrist Surg 2018;7(1):38–42.

40. Morgan WJ, Breen TF, Coumas JM, et al. Role of magnetic resonance imaging in assessing factors affecting healing in scaphoid nonunions. Clin Orthop Relat Res 1997;336:240–6.

41. Bush CH, Gillespy T 3rd, Dell PC. High-resolution CT of the wrist: initial experience with scaphoid disorders and surgical fusions. AJR Am J Roentgenol 1987;149(4):757–60.

42. Drijkoningen T, Ten Berg PWL, Guitton TG, et al. Reliability of diagnosis of partial union of scaphoid waist fractures on computed tomography. J Hand Microsurg 2018;10(3):130–3.

43. Ganapathi M, Joseph G, Savage R, et al. MRI susceptibility artefacts related to scaphoid screws: the effect of screw type, screw orientation and imaging parameters. J Hand Surg Br 2002;27(2):165–70.

44. Downing ND, Oni JA, Davis TR, et al. The relationship between proximal pole blood flow and the subjective assessment of increased density of the proximal pole in acute scaphoid fractures. J Hand Surg Am 2002;27(3):402–8.

45. Pianta M, McCombe D, Slavin J, et al. Dual-energy contrast-enhanced CT to evaluate scaphoid osteonecrosis with surgical correlation. J Med Imaging Radiat Oncol 2019;63(1):69–75.

46. Ten Berg PWL, de Roo MGA, Maas M, et al. Is there a trend in CT scanning scaphoid nonunions for deformity assessment?-A systematic review. Eur J Radiol 2017;91:124–9.

47. Ten Berg PW, Dobbe JG, Horbach SE, et al. Analysis of deformity in scaphoid non-unions using two- and three-dimensional imaging. J Hand Surg Eur Vol 2016;41(7):719–26.

48. Megerle K, Harenberg PS, Germann G, et al. Scaphoid morphology and clinical outcomes in scaphoid reconstructions. Injury 2012;43(3):306–10.

49. ten Berg PW, Dobbe JG, Strackee SD, et al. Three-dimensional assessment of bilateral symmetry of the scaphoid: an anatomic study. Biomed Res Int 2015;2015:547250.

50. McNally EG, Goodman R, Burge P. The role of MRI in the assessment of scaphoid fracture healing: a pilot study. Eur Radiol 2000;10(12):1926–8.

51. Dawson JS, Martel AL, Davis TR. Scaphoid blood flow and acute fracture healing. A dynamic MRI study with enhancement with gadolinium. J Bone Joint Surg Br 2001;83(6):809–14.

52. Trumble TE. Avascular necrosis after scaphoid fracture: a correlation of magnetic resonance imaging and histology. J Hand Surg Am 1990;15(4):557–64.

53. Fox MG, Gaskin CM, Chhabra AB, et al. Assessment of scaphoid viability with MRI: a reassessment of findings on unenhanced MR images. AJR Am J Roentgenol 2010;195(4):W281–6.

54. Donati OF, Zanetti M, Nagy L, et al. Is dynamic gadolinium enhancement needed in MR imaging for the preoperative assessment of scaphoidal viability in patients with scaphoid nonunion? Radiology 2011;260(3):808–16.

55. Werneck L, Canella C, Costa F, et al. Usefulness of dynamic contrast-enhanced MRI in the evaluation of osteonecrosis of the proximal fragment in scaphoid fractures. Radiol Bras 2018;51(5):334.

56. Ng AW, Griffith JF, Taljanovic MS, et al. Is dynamic contrast-enhanced MRI useful for assessing proximal fragment vascularity in scaphoid fracture delayed and non-union? Skeletal Radiol 2013;42(7):983–92.

57. Larribe M, Gay A, Freire V, et al. Usefulness of dynamic contrast-enhanced MRI in the evaluation of the viability of acute scaphoid fracture. Skeletal Radiol 2014;43(12):1697–703.

58. Fox MG, Wang DT, Chhabra AB. Accuracy of enhanced and unenhanced MRI in diagnosing scaphoid proximal pole avascular necrosis and predicting surgical outcome. Skeletal Radiol 2015;44(11):1671–8.

59. Anderson SE, Steinbach LS, Tschering-Vogel D, et al. MR imaging of avascular scaphoid nonunion before and after vascularized bone grafting. Skeletal Radiol 2005;34(6):314–20.

60. Dailiana ZH, Zachos V, Varitimidis S, et al. Scaphoid nonunions treated with vascularised bone grafts: MRI assessment. Eur J Radiol 2004;50(3):217–24.

61. Houdek MT, Matsumoto JM, Morris JM, et al. Technique for 3-dimesional (3D) modeling of osteoarticular medial femoral condyle vascularized grafting to replace the proximal pole of unsalvagable scaphoid nonunions. Tech Hand Up Extrem Surg 2016;20(3):117–24.

62. Yamabe E, Anavim A, Sakai T, et al. Comparison between high-resolution isotropic three-dimensional and high-resolution conventional two-dimensional FSE MR images of the wrist at 3 tesla: a pilot study. J Magn Reson Imaging 2014;40(3):603–8.

63. Stevens KJ, Wallace CG, Chen W, et al. Imaging of the wrist at 1.5 Tesla using isotropic three-dimensional fast spin echo cube. J Magn Reson Imaging 2011;33(4):908–15.

64. Ten Berg PWL, Dobbe JGG, Streekstra GJ. Short report letter: three-dimensional printed anatomical models in scaphoid surgery. J Hand Surg Eur Vol 2018;43(1):101–2.

65. Mitsouras D, Liacouras P, Imanzadeh A, et al. Medical 3D printing for the radiologist. Radiographics 2015;35(7):1965–88.

66. George E, Liacouras P, Rybicki FJ, et al. Measuring and establishing the accuracy and reproducibility of 3D printed medical models. Radiographics 2017; 37(5):1424–50.

Diagnosis and Management of Acute Scaphoid Fractures

M. Diya Sabbagh, MBBS[a,b], Mohamed Morsy, MB, BCh[b,c],
Steven L. Moran, MD[a],*

KEYWORDS

- Scaphoid • Scaphoid fracture • Dorsal approach • Compression screw • Wrist

KEY POINTS

- Scaphoid fractures are the most common carpal bone fracture, and 10% to 15% may present with normal radiographs.
- Computed tomography (CT) or MRI remain the best means of ruling out a fracture, whereas CT remains the best means of determining scaphoid displacement.
- Surgical management with a compression screw may be a more cost-effective means of treating fractures, but is associated with higher complication rates for nondisplaced waist fractures.
- A percutaneous dorsal approach allows for a safe and reliable means of treating minimally displaced fractures.

▶ Video content accompanies this article at http://www.hand.theclinics.com.

INTRODUCTION

The scaphoid is an obliquely oriented bone located on the radial side of the wrist. It is an important carpal bone, bridging the proximal and distal carpal rows. The scaphoid contributes significantly to the wrist stability and biomechanical function, because its motion has an impact on the motion of the lunate (through its attachment of the scapholunate interosseous ligament) and the motion of the distal carpal row. The scaphoid is mainly intraarticular, and 80% of the bone is covered by cartilage forming an articular surface. Most of the proximal one-half of the scaphoid is covered with articular cartilage. This allows for only a small surface area for vascular inflow. The scaphoid's arterial foramina span the nonarticulating palmar and dorsal surface. The bone receives its blood supply through its ligamentous attachments. Studies by Gelberman and Menon[1] have shown that in 75% of scaphoid specimens, 2 arteries branch off the radial artery to supply the scaphoid on the dorsal and proximal surfaces; these branches are the dorsal carpal branch and the superficial palmar branch, respectively. In 20% of scaphoids, most of the arterial foramina exist in the waist area. Because of this arterial interosseous anatomy, the articular proximal pole of the scaphoid receives its blood supply in a retrograde fashion, hence this may explain the high incidence of proximal pole avascular necrosis and nonunion in untreated fractures involving this region[2,3] (Fig. 1).

Among carpal bone injuries, scaphoid fractures are considered the most common with an estimated incidence ranging from 50% to 70% of all

[a] Division of Plastic and Reconstructive Surgery, Department of Surgery, Mayo Clinic, 200 1st Street Southwest, Rochester, MN 55902, USA; [b] Division of Plastic Surgery, Mayo 12, 200 First Street Southwest, Rochester, MN 55905, USA; [c] Department of Orthopedic Surgery, Assiut University Hospital, Assiut University, Assiut, Egypt
* Corresponding author.
E-mail address: Moran.Steven@Mayo.edu

Hand Clin 35 (2019) 259–269
https://doi.org/10.1016/j.hcl.2019.03.002

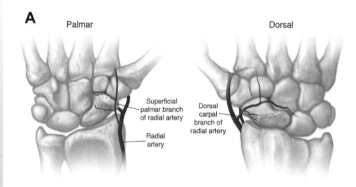

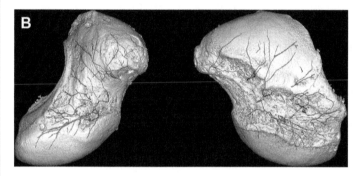

Fig. 1. (*A*) Scaphoid blood supply. Most of the blood flow enters the scaphoid distally at the level of the dorsal ridge and through the proximal tubercle. Hence, fractures of the proximal pole may leave a segment of proximal bone with poor intrinsic blood supply and at risk of nonunion and avascular necrosis. (*B*) A 3-dimensional micro-computed tomography (micro-CT) reconstruction of a CT showing the interosseous blood supply entering the scaphoid. (Used with permission of Mayo Foundation for Medical Education and Research, all rights reserved.)

carpal bone fractures and up to 11% of all hand fractures. Scaphoid fractures occur more commonly in younger men.[4–7] Van Tassel and colleagues,[7] using the National Electronic Injury Surveillance System database, found the incidence to be 1.47 per 100,000 person-years. This incidence of fracture may be higher in athletes and military personnel.[8,9] In children, scaphoid fractures are less common, accounting for only 3% of all fractures of the pediatric hand and wrist.[10–12] The thick peripheral cartilage that covers the scaphoid and protects the ossification center may explain the lower incidence of scaphoid fractures in children.

Despite their frequency, acute scaphoid fractures can go unrecognized or be misdiagnosed as a wrist "sprain." Presenting symptoms may be minimal and initial radiographs can be negative for fracture. Unfortunately, delays in treatment can lead to malunion, nonunion, or avascular necrosis.[13–15] All 3 of these problems create increasing complexity for surgical correction. Neglected scaphoid fractures will progress to a predictable pattern of wrist arthritis know as scaphoid nonunion advanced collapse arthritis (**Fig. 2**). Thus, early diagnosis and proper management are crucial to ensure preservation of the wrist function and kinematics.[16–20] This article reviews the diagnosis and management of acute scaphoid fractures.

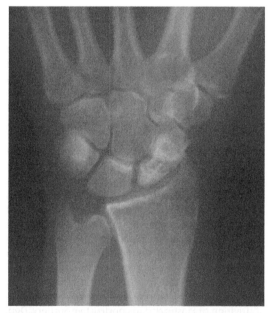

Fig. 2. Anteroposterior (AP) radiograph showing evidence of a scaphoid nonunion, which has progressed to scaphoid nonunion advanced collapse (SNAC) arthritis. Joint narrowing can be seen along the radial styloid and the joint surface between the scaphoid and capitate.

MECHANISM OF INJURY

Scaphoid fractures most commonly result from a fall on an outstretched hand with the wrist in extension and radial deviation.[13,21] The exact biomechanical mechanism of the fracture has been debatable. Todd was the first to study the mechanism of scaphoid fractures and he believed that they occur due to excessive tension,[22] whereas Cobey and White argued that scaphoid fractures result from excessive compression along the scaphoid's concave medial articulation surface with the capitate.[23] In a cadaveric study, Frykman demonstrated that scaphoid fractures are more likely to occur with hyperextension of the wrist with radial deviation.[24] Weber and Chao further confirmed the aforementioned findings and were able to create scaphoid fractures by having a load applied to the radial portion of the palm with the wrist in only 95° to 100° extension.[20,25,26] Most of the fractures affect the middle third of the scaphoid.[27]

Scaphoid fractures may also occur concomitantly with other injuries and one should have a high index of suspicion for distal radius fractures and associated perilunate injury patterns in cases of higher velocity trauma. Variations in the classic ligamentous pattern of perilunate injury can occur, resulting in associated fractures of carpal bones. Areas of potential fracture include the distal radius, scaphoid, trapezium, capitate, hamate, and triquetrum, although the scaphoid is the most common. All fractures are aligned along a larger arc encircling the lunate (**Fig. 3**). The term "greater arc injury" refers to any perilunate injury pattern involving bony fracture through this greater arc, whereas the term "lesser arc injury" describes a pattern of pure ligamentous disruption, which follows a smaller arc immediately around the lunate.[28] In the descriptive nomenclature, the prefix "trans" is used to denote the fractured bone or bones (ie, "transscaphoid dorsal perilunate dislocation") (see **Fig. 3**B).

DIAGNOSIS

A high degree of clinical suspicion is important to avoid missing a minimally displaced fracture. A scaphoid fracture should be suspected in any young patient with a fall on outstretched hand or an injury with the wrist in dorsiflexion. Patients present with wrist pain, but pain can be minimal. The classic clinical signs include tenderness with palpation over the anatomic snuff box and scaphoid tubercle, in addition to pain with axial compression of the thumb (referred to as the compression test).[29,30] Tenderness over the

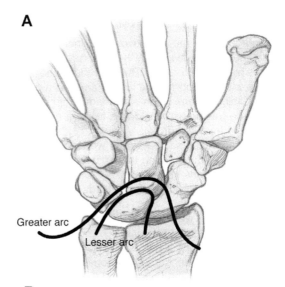

A

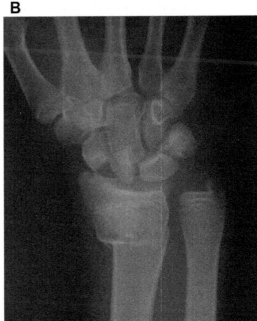

B

Fig. 3. (A) A potential greater arc injury pattern. During a perilunate injury, a pure ligamentous injury can occur (lesser arc injury) or an injury that results in a fracture dislocation pattern may occur (greater arc injury). (B) AP radiograph of a transscaphoid dorsal perilunate fracture dislocation with associated distal radius fracture in a skeletally immature patient. ([A] Used with permission of Mayo Foundation for Medical Education and Research, all rights reserved.)

anatomic snuff box suggests scaphoid fracture until proved otherwise.[31] Four views of the wrist are considered the standard to evaluate a possible scaphoid fracture; these include a posteroanterior view with ulnar deviation of the wrist, lateral, semi-pronated oblique, and semisupinated oblique.[32]

Adequate initial radiographs detect fractures in 85% to 90% of the cases[33,34]; however, initial radiographs may be negative. The incidence of false-negative radiographs has been reported to be as high as 25%.[14,34,35] Thus, a patient who presents with the appropriate history and has a positive clinical examination with radiographs that show no fracture is considered to have a clinical scaphoid fracture (**Fig. 4**).

Clinical scaphoid fractures were historically managed by immobilizing the wrist and repeating plain radiographs in 3 weeks.[36–42] The disadvantage of this approach is that it leads to unnecessary immobilization, loss of productivity, and income. This 3-week time delay can be removed because present day imaging modalities are more reliable than plain radiographs.[14,43–45] These modalities include computed tomography (CT), MRI, bone scans, and ultrasound (US).

US screening and evaluation for scaphoid fracture is an attractive alternative to CT and radiographs, because US is prevalent in most medical practices, avoid radiation, and can be performed quickly within an emergency room or office setting. Recently Jain and colleagues[46] showed, in a prospective study of 114 patients, that the accuracy of detecting a scaphoid fracture with US was 98% in comparison to radiographs that were only positive 20% of the time. Although these values need to be corroborated with other studies, this may provide an easy means of screening clinical scaphoid fractures.

Despite the potential importance of US in diagnosing acute fractures, MRI remains the most useful imaging modality to detect hidden fractures, because edema within the bone can be detected on MRI within hours of injury.[47] Another advantage is that MRI can detect other coexisting ligamentous and wrist injuries. Several studies have showed that MRI is an appropriate second-line study in detecting acute scaphoid fractures with a sensitivity and specificity approaching 100%.[14,41,48–51] Both high-resolution CT scans and bone scan seem to be a good alternative in patients who cannot undergo MRI. Bone scan has the highest sensitivity but it has a low specificity. CT scan has 72% sensitivity and 99% specificity.[45] It is important to keep in mind that although bone scans are statistically the best diagnostic modality to establish a definitive diagnosis, they are more invasive and associated with more radiation exposure than other studies.[45,52,53] At the authors' institution, patients who have positive clinical findings that suggest scaphoid fractures with equivocal plain radiographs undergo immediate MRI or CT scans. Repeat radiographs are also obtained at 2 to 3 weeks.

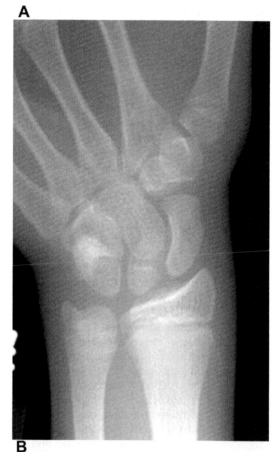

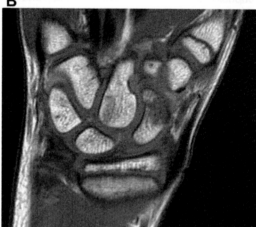

Fig. 4. A 12-year-old boy with pain in the snuff box following a fall onto wrist. (*A*) Initial radiographs were read as normal. (*B*) The adolescent was splinted and sent for MRI, which revealed a distal pole scaphoid fracture.

MANAGEMENT

Optimal treatment and management of scaphoid fractures depends on the timing (early or late presentation), appropriate diagnosis, and the type of the fracture. Delays in treatment increase the risk of nonunion and the need for surgical management. Langhoff and Andersen demonstrated that when treatment is delayed by 4 weeks, the risk of nonunion can be as high as 40%, a significant increased risk when compared with the 3% risk of nonunion when diagnosis and treatment occurred within 4 weeks.[54–56] Even problematic proximal pole fractures have been reported to have an acceptable rate of union if treated within 4 weeks of injury.[57,58]

In addition to time to treatment, several other factors are thought to contribute to nonunion and complications; these factors include the degree of fracture displacement, location of the fracture, and fracture stability. Scaphoid fractures can be classified according to their anatomic location and stability. Herbert, in his classic description, proposed an alpha-numeric classification system that combines fracture anatomy, stability, and history (**Fig. 5**). The classification system provides a grade with prognostic significance.[59,60] Oka and Morimoto have shown that fractures occurring distal to the apex of the dorsal scaphoid ridge (Herbert B2) are more likely to proceed to collapse and humpback deformity due to the

loss ligamentous stability on the distal fragment.[61,62] The ability to distinguish unstable from stable fractures is essential, because it determines who needs surgical management.[54,63]

Conservative, Nonsurgical Treatment

Immobilization remains an acceptable option for managing stable, nondisplaced fractures; these include nondisplaced waist and distal pole fractures.[64] Cooney and colleagues[65] defined displacement as a fracture gap of 1 mm or less on anteroposterior and oblique radiographs; a lunate-capitate angle is less than 15° and the scapholunate angle is no more than 60° in the lateral view. To accurately judge displacement, it is recommended to obtain a CT on all fractures; furthermore, recent evidence suggests that 3-dimensional CT scans may be the best means of determining fracture type and stability.[61]

If the fracture is a mid-waist or distal pole fracture, stable and nondisplaced casting is an appropriate treatment; however, the extent of joint immobilization (thumb, wrist, and/or forearm) to obtain successful union has been an issue of historic debate. Cadaveric studies have shown

TYPE A:
STABLE ACUTE FRACTURES

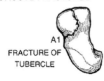
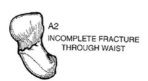

A1
FRACTURE OF TUBERCLE

A2
INCOMPLETE FRACTURE THROUGH WAIST

Fig. 5. Herbert classification scheme for scaphoid fractures. (*From* Herbert TJ. The fractured scaphoid. St Louis: Quality Medical Publishing; 1990; with permission.)

TYPE B:
UNSTABLE ACUTE FRACTURES

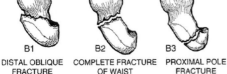
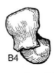

B1
DISTAL OBLIQUE FRACTURE

B2
COMPLETE FRACTURE OF WAIST

B3
PROXIMAL POLE FRACTURE

B4
TRANS-SCAPHOID-PERILUNATE FRACTURE DISLOCATION OF CARPUS

TYPE C:
DELAYED UNION

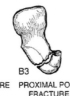

C
DELAYED UNION

TYPE D:
ESTABLISHED NONUNION

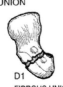
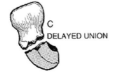
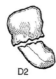

D1
FIBROUS UNION

D2
PSEUDARTHROSIS

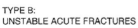

evidence of displacement of the proximal and distal poles within simulated scaphoid fractures as the arm moves between pronation and supination.[66] Despite these cadaveric studies, current meta-analysis and systemic reviews have failed to show any significant benefit of immobilization of the forearm, elbow, or thumb.[67] Thus, immobilization need only be performed distal to the elbow with the wrist in the functional position. Clay and colleagues[68] found no benefit to immobilization of the thumb or elbow almost 3 decades ago. In a recent multicenter randomized controlled trial, Buijze and colleagues[69] examined 62 patients and found that immobilization of the thumb is unnecessary for cases of CT-confirmed nondisplaced or minimally displaced fractures of the waist of the scaphoid.

Studies have shown that nondisplaced fractures of the waist can heal in 8 weeks in 90% of the cases with appropriate immobilization.[65,70–73] This success rate argues for nonoperative management in most of the nondisplaced stable waist fractures; however, the argument for early operative intervention has been shown to decrease overall cost and result in decrease immobilization times.[51,74] A recent meta-analysis showed operative fixation to result in better motion, decreased rates of delayed union, and decreased time away from work.[75] Davis and colleagues[76] using a decision-based model found that when compared with casting, open reduction and internal fixation offered a cost-saving. Despite these benefits, randomized series as well as meta-analysis have shown that surgical treatment is associated with more risk and complications.[20,77,78] Long-term risks and benefits of surgical intervention should be carefully weighed and considered when deciding on how to best manage a stable waist fracture.

Surgical Management

Surgical management is indicated for unstable fractures, proximal pole fractures, displaced waist fractures, and fractures where the gap is more than 1 mm.[65] As mentioned earlier, the proximal pole has a limited blood supply, which explains the high incidence of nonunion and the necessity of surgical management.[57] Humpback deformity is also an indication for surgery. In cases of large fragments, headless compression screws are the most common means of fixation. In cases where the proximal fragment is too small to accept a screw, Kirschner wires (K-wire) can be used to reduce and stabilize the fracture.[79,80] The benefits of newer scaphoid plates and double screw fixation have yet to be determined. Historically,

excellent results have been reported for open surgical approaches using compression screws, with both Dias and Trumble reporting union rates of 100%.[70,81]

Open techniques can result in disruption of the scaphoid's blood supply as well as capsular scaring, which may limit postoperative motion. Because of the associated morbidity with open surgical approaches, most acute fractures can now be reduced and treated through a percutaneous or arthroscopic assisted approach, even when bone grafting is required.[82,83] Despite the success of percutaneous techniques, patients should be aware that in cases where percutaneous fixation fails or fracture reduction is not adequate, a conversion to an open surgery will be needed.[81]

Regardless of the type of approach used, it is important to obtain a good entry point through the proximal or distal fragment during screw placement. Studies by Dodds and colleagues[84] and McCallister and colleagues[85] have demonstrated that a centrally placed screw provides 43% greater stiffness and 39% increased load to failure when compared with an eccentrically placed screws. Central placement is found to be achieved more consistently with cannulated screws.[86,87] In addition, the screw should be positioned at a right angle to the fracture line if possible. Thus, the type and location of the fracture dictates the preference for a volar or dorsal approach. Most B1 and B2 fractures can be managed through a dorsal approach, whereas correction of humpback deformity usually requires a volar approach. Volar approaches are at increased risk of scaphotrapeziotrapezoidal arthritis, whereas the dorsal approach places the extensor pollicis longus (EPL) tendon at risk of injury.[88] A recent meta-analysis comparing the dorsal to the volar approach was performed by Kang and colleagues.[89] The study found no difference between the incidence of nonunion, complications, postoperative pain, functional outcome, or grip strength when comparing the volar with dorsal screw placement. Although no benefit has been clearly shown, surgeons should be familiar with each approach.

Dorsal miniopen approach and percutaneous fixation

The authors prefer to perform a percutaneous fixation of the scaphoid via a mini-open dorsal approach for Herbert B1 or B2 fractures (Video 1). To begin the procedure, Lister's tubercle is marked along with the radial styloid. The scapholunate ligament usually lies just ulnar and distal to the tubercle. It is important to keep in mind that the waist of scaphoid lays at the intersection of the

EPL and the extensor carpi radialis brevis (ECRB) tendons. A 1 to 1.5 cm incision is made lateral to the Lister's tubercle to allow for safe placement of a KirsK-wire and identification and protection of the EPL tendon. Meticulous dissection should be done until the EPL and ECRB are identified. The K-wire may now be pushed manually through the dorsal wrist capsule to abut the proximal dorsal scaphoid surface. The wrist is now flexed approximately 45o and thumb is then distracted in 45° of palmar and radial abduction. The K-wire is directed through the scaphoid toward the thumb tip. This K-wire will be used for guidance before drilling. If difficulty is encountered in finding the central axis of the scaphoid during guidewire placement, intraoperative fluoroscopy may be used to facilitate placement.

Although the authors prefer the technique described earlier for obtaining the central axis for K-wire positioning, the technique described by

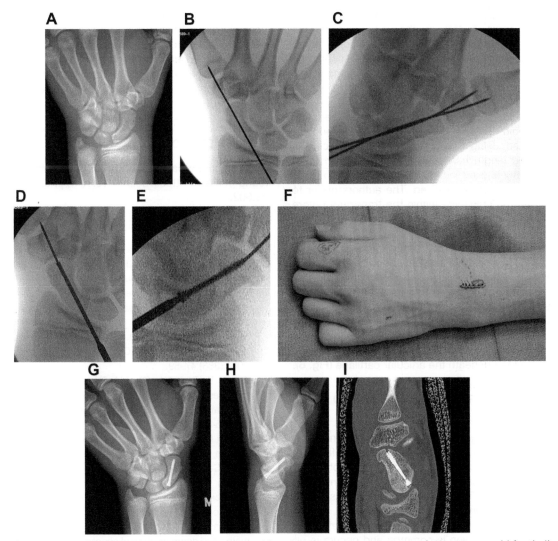

Fig. 6. A case of a scaphoid waist fracture treated with a dorsal percutaneous approach in a 16-year-old football player. (*A*) Ulnar deviated scaphoid view showing minimally displaced left scaphoid fracture. (*B*) Central placement of the K-wire is critical for central screw placement. (*C*) A second K-wire is placed as an antirotational wire, before reaming the scaphoid. (*D*) Reaming is performed with the aid of the fluoroscanner to prevent over drilling. (*E*) A compression screw has been placed across the fracture site. An oblique view is helpful to prevent screw placement into the scaphotrapeziotrapezoid joint. (*F*) Appearance of the hand at completion of the case. The mini-open approach allows for protection of the EPL and ECRB tendons during screw placement. (*G, H*) AP and lateral radiographs showing healed fracture and good carpal alignment. (*I*) Final CT showing complete healing and a well-positioned screw at 8 weeks.

Slade may also be used.[82,90] The central axis of the scaphoid is identified by flexing and pronating the wrist, at which point the scaphoid, through the fluoroscanner, will appear as a cylinder. By aligning the K-wire directly with the proximal pole of the scaphoid, the center portion of the cylinder is targeted and the K-wires then driven out through the base of the trapezium. At this point the wire can be withdrawn through the palm until it clears the radial carpal joint; the wrist can then be extended and the position of the wire examined before placing a self-compression screw.

Once the K-wire location is confirmed using a fluoroscopic C-arm in the long axis of the scaphoid, an antirotational wire is placed before reaming over the guidewire. The screw should be introduced near the scapholunate ligament and not through the dorsal portion of the bone to ensure central axial placement within the scaphoid. It is important not to over-ream the scaphoid. The depth of the drill is continuously checked using the fluroscanner and once the desired length has been reached, a cannulated obturator is used to hold the guide K-wire in place as the drill bit is removed. The authors prefer to imbed the guidewire within the trapezium before reaming to prevent guidewire displacement during drill removal.

The drill bit is subsequently removed by hand carefully to avoid displacement of the guide K-wire. The needed screw length can be measured preoperatively or intraoperatively using screw measurement system to obtain the appropriate screw length, which is usually 28 to 24 mm. We always subtract at least 4 mm from the scaphoid length, so the screw may be safely embedded beneath the articular cartilage (**Fig. 6**).

IDENTIFYING UNION AND RETURN TO ACTIVITY

Union is an ongoing process rather than an occurrence at a point of time. Nonunion is defined as absence of signs of healing on radiographs after 12 weeks of management and the presence of a clear gap on CT scans or MRI. Union is assessed by serial imaging and clinical observation, but the authors rely on CT scan to definitively determine union. Partial union is common and occurs in up to 40% of cases.[91–95]

Return to activity depends on the patient characteristics and the type of the fracture; thus, the decision on when to resume normal activities should be personalized to each patient. Brekke and colleagues[96] noted that inherent stability of the scaphoid was maintained with at least 25% scaphoid waist intact. The authors' protocol is usually to wait for evidence of union in 50% of the fracture and evidence of a firmly seated screw. The risk of refracture is high, and patients are generally advised to refrain from participating in contact sports for 2 to 3 months following healing; this can be especially challenging in competitive athletes. Playing casts, which are generally softer and lighter, can be used during games to protect both the patient and other players from injury. Soft casts were not found to influence the outcome or delay healing.[97] Competitive athletes and sports players whose careers are at stake should be encouraged to return to play as soon as it is safely possible. Other patients who are recreational athletes should be treated more cautiously. All of the aforementioned should be discussed thoroughly with the patient to ensure that they are aware of the management plan, risk or reinjury, and reasonable expectations on recovery.[98]

SUPPLEMENTARY DATA

Supplementary data related to this article can be found online at https://doi.org/10.1016/j.hcl.2019.03.002.

REFERENCES

1. Gelberman RH, Menon J. The vascularity of the scaphoid bone. J Hand Surg Am 1980;5(5):508–13.
2. Botte MJ, Pacelli LL, Gelberman RH. Vascularity and osteonecrosis of the wrist. Orthop Clin North Am 2004;35(3):405–21, xi.
3. Freedman DM, Botte MJ, Gelberman RH. Vascularity of the carpus. Clin Orthop Relat Res 2001;(383):47–59.
4. Garala K, Taub NA, Dias JJ. The epidemiology of fractures of the scaphoid: impact of age, gender, deprivation and seasonality. Bone Joint J 2016;98-B(5):654–9.
5. Hove LM. Epidemiology of scaphoid fractures in Bergen, Norway. Scand J Plast Reconstr Surg Hand Surg 1999;33(4):423–6.
6. Larsen CF, Brondum V, Skov O. Epidemiology of scaphoid fractures in Odense, Denmark. Acta Orthop Scand 1992;63(2):216–8.
7. Van Tassel DC, Owens BD, Wolf JM. Incidence estimates and demographics of scaphoid fracture in the U.S. population. J Hand Surg Am 2010;35(8):1242–5.
8. Winston MJ, Weiland AJ. Scaphoid fractures in the athlete. Curr Rev Musculoskelet Med 2017;10(1):38–44.
9. Wolf JM, Dawson L, Mountcastle SB, et al. The incidence of scaphoid fracture in a military population. Injury 2009;40(12):1316–9.

10. Mussbichler H. Injuries of the carpal scaphoid in children. Acta Radiol 1961;56:361–8.

11. Kocher MS, Waters PM, Micheli LJ. Upper extremity injuries in the paediatric athlete. Sports Med 2000; 30(2):117–35.

12. Elhassan BT, Shin AY. Scaphoid fracture in children. Hand Clin 2006;22(1):31–41.

13. Kozin SH. Incidence, mechanism, and natural history of scaphoid fractures. Hand Clin 2001;17(4): 515–24.

14. Jenkins PJ, Slade K, Huntley JS, et al. A comparative analysis of the accuracy, diagnostic uncertainty and cost of imaging modalities in suspected scaphoid fractures. Injury 2008;39(7):768–74.

15. Rhemrev SJ, Beeres FJ, van Leerdam RH, et al. Clinical prediction rule for suspected scaphoid fractures: a prospective cohort study. Injury 2010; 41(10):1026–30.

16. Amadio PC, Berquist TH, Smith DK, et al. Scaphoid malunion. J Hand Surg 1989;14A:679–87.

17. Fernandez DL, Eggli S. Scaphoid nonunion and malunion. How to correct deformity. Hand Clin 2001; 17(4):631–46, ix.

18. Lee CH, Lee KH, Lee BG, et al. Clinical outcome of scaphoid malunion as a result of scaphoid fracture nonunion surgical treatment: a 5-year minimum follow-up study. Orthop Traumatol Surg Res 2015; 101(3):359–63.

19. Janowski J, Coady C, Catalano LW 3rd. Scaphoid fractures: nonunion and malunion. J Hand Surg Am 2016;41(11):1087–92.

20. Ibrahim T, Qureshi A, Sutton AJ, et al. Surgical versus nonsurgical treatment of acute minimally displaced and undisplaced scaphoid waist fractures: pairwise and network meta-analyses of randomized controlled trials. J Hand Surg Am 2011;36(11): 1759–68.e1.

21. Mayfield JK. Mechanism of carpal injuries. Clin Orthop Relat Res 1980;(149):45–54.

22. Todd AH. Fractures of the carpal scaphoid. Br J Surg 1921;9:7–26.

23. Cobey MC, White RK. An operation for non-union of fractures of the carpal navicular. J Bone Joint Surg Am 1946;28(4):757–64.

24. Frykman G. Fracture of the distal radius including sequelae–shoulder-hand-finger syndrome, disturbance in the distal radio-ulnar joint and impairment of nerve function. A clinical and experimental study. Acta Orthop Scand 1967;(Suppl 108):3+.

25. Weber ER. Biomechanical implications of scaphoid waist fractures. Clin Orthop 1980;149:83–9.

26. Weber ER, Chao EYS. An experimental approach to the mechanism of scaphoid waist fractures. J Hand Surg 1978;3:142–8.

27. Polsky MB, Kozin SH, Porter ST, et al. Scaphoid fractures: dorsal versus volar approach. Orthopedics 2002;25(8):817–9.

28. Chim H, Moran SL. Wrist essentials: the diagnosis and management of scapholunate ligament injuries. Plast Reconstr Surg 2014;134(2):312e–22e.

29. Parvizi J, Wayman J, Kelly P, et al. Combining the clinical signs improves diagnosis of scaphoid fractures. A prospective study with follow-up. J Hand Surg Br 1998;23(3):324–7.

30. Grover R. Clinical assessment of scaphoid injuries and the detection of fractures. J Hand Surg Br 1996;21(3):341–3.

31. Watson-Jones R. The classic: "fractures and joint injuries" by Sir Reginald Watson-Jones, taken from "fractures and joint injuries," by R. Watson-Jones, vol. II, 4th ed., Baltimore, Williams and Wilkins Company, 1955. Clin Orthop Relat Res 1974;(105):4–10.

32. Compson JP, Waterman JK, Heatley FW. The radiological anatomy of the scaphoid. Part 2: radiology. J Hand Surg Br 1997;22(1):8–15.

33. Hunter JC, Escobedo EM, Wilson AJ, et al. MR imaging of clinically suspected scaphoid fractures. AJR Am J Roentgenol 1997;168(5):1287–93.

34. Leslie IJ, Dickson RA. The fractured carpal scaphoid. Natural history and factors influencing outcome. J Bone Joint Surg Br 1981;63-B(2): 225–30.

35. Waeckerle JF. A prospective study identifying the sensitivity of radiographic findings and the efficacy of clinical findings in carpal navicular fractures. Ann Emerg Med 1987;16(7):733–7.

36. Sjolin SU, Andersen JC. Clinical fracture of the carpal scaphoid–supportive bandage or plaster cast immobilization? J Hand Surg Br 1988;13(1):75–6.

37. DaCruz DJ, Bodiwala GG, Finlay DB. The suspected fracture of the scaphoid: a rational approach to diagnosis. Injury 1988;19(3):149–52.

38. Hill NA. Fractures and dislocations of the carpus. Orthop Clin North Am 1970;1(2):275–84.

39. Russe O. Fracture of the carpal navicular. Diagnosis, non-operative treatment, and operative treatment. J Bone Joint Surg Am 1960;42-A:759–68.

40. Brydie A, Raby N. Early MRI in the management of clinical scaphoid fracture. Br J Radiol 2003; 76(905):296–300.

41. Shetty S, Sidharthan S, Jacob J, et al. 'Clinical scaphoid fracture': is it time to abolish this phrase? Ann R Coll Surg Engl 2011;93(2):146–8.

42. Rhemrev SJ, van Leerdam RH, Beeres FJ, et al. Bone scintigraphy in patients with clinical suspicion of a scaphoid fracture. Eur J Emerg Med 2010;17(2): 124–5.

43. Yin ZG, Zhang JB, Kan SL, et al. Diagnosing suspected scaphoid fractures: a systematic review and meta-analysis. Clin Orthop Relat Res 2010; 468(3):723–34.

44. Nichols AW. Comparison of imaging techniques for diagnosing suspected scaphoid fractures: a review. Clin J Sport Med 2010;20(5):393–4.

45. Mallee WH, Wang J, Poolman RW, et al. Computed tomography versus magnetic resonance imaging versus bone scintigraphy for clinically suspected scaphoid fractures in patients with negative plain radiographs. Cochrane Database Syst Rev 2015;(6): CD010023.

46. Jain R, Jain N, Sheikh T, et al. Early scaphoid fractures are better diagnosed with ultrasonography than X-rays: a prospective study over 114 patients. Chin J Traumatol 2018;21(4):206–10.

47. Adams JE, Steinmann SP. Acute scaphoid fractures. Hand Clin 2010;26(1):97–103.

48. Memarsadeghi M, Breitenseher MJ, Schaefer-Prokop C, et al. Occult scaphoid fractures: comparison of multidetector CT and MR imaging–initial experience. Radiology 2006;240(1):169–76.

49. Foex B, Speake P, Body R. Best evidence topic report. Magnetic resonance imaging or bone scintigraphy in the diagnosis of plain x ray occult scaphoid fractures. Emerg Med J 2005;22(6):434–5.

50. Patel NK, Davies N, Mirza Z, et al. Cost and clinical effectiveness of MRI in occult scaphoid fractures: a randomised controlled trial. Emerg Med J 2013; 30(3):202–7.

51. Arsalan-Werner A, Sauerbier M, Mehling IM. Current concepts for the treatment of acute scaphoid fractures. Eur J Trauma Emerg Surg 2016;42(1): 3–10.

52. Tiel-van Buul MM, Broekhuizen TH, van Beek EJ, et al. Choosing a strategy for the diagnostic management of suspected scaphoid fracture: a cost-effectiveness analysis. J Nucl Med 1995;36(1): 45–8.

53. Yin ZG, Zhang JB, Gong KT. Cost-effectiveness of diagnostic strategies for suspected scaphoid fractures. J Orthop Trauma 2015;29(8):e245–52.

54. Wong K, von Schroeder HP. Delays and poor management of scaphoid fractures: factors contributing to nonunion. J Hand Surg Am 2011;36(9):1471–4.

55. Langhoff O, Andersen JL. Consequences of late immobilization of scaphoid fractures. J Hand Surg Br 1988;13(1):77–9.

56. Eddeland A, Eiken O, Hellgren E, et al. Fractures of the scaphoid. Scand J Plast Reconstr Surg 1975; 9(3):234–9.

57. Brogan DM, Moran SL, Shin AY. Outcomes of open reduction and internal fixation of acute proximal pole scaphoid fractures. Hand (N Y) 2015;10(2): 227–32.

58. Retting ME, Raskin KB. Retrograde compression screw fixation of acute proximal pole scaphoid fractures. J Hand Surg 1999;24A:1206–10.

59. Herbert TJ. The fractured scaphoid. St Louis (MO): Quality Medical Publishing; 1990.

60. Krimmer H, Lanz U. Post-traumatic carpal collapse. Follow-up and therapeutic concept. Unfallchirurg 2000;103(4):260–6 [in German].

61. Oka K, Moritomo H. Current management of scaphoid nonunion based on the biomechanical study. J Wrist Surg 2017;7(2):94–100.

62. Moritomo H, Viegas SF, Elder KW, et al. Scaphoid nonunions: a three-dimensional analysis of paterns of deformity. J Hand Surg 2000;25:520–8.

63. Ferguson DO, Shanbhag V, Hedley H, et al. Scaphoid fracture non-union: a systematic review of surgical treatment using bone graft. J Hand Surg Eur Vol 2016;41(5):492–500.

64. Tada K, Ikeda K, Okamoto S, et al. Scaphoid fracture–overview and conservative treatment. Hand Surg 2015;20(2):204–9.

65. Cooney WP, Dobyns JH, Linscheid RL. Fractures of the scaphoid: a rational approach to management. Clin Orthop 1980;149:90–7.

66. Kaneshiro SA, Failla JM, Tashman S. Scaphoid fracture displacement with forearm rotation in a short-arm thumb spica cast. J Hand Surg 1999;24A(5): 984–91.

67. Doornberg JN, Buijze GA, Ham SJ, et al. Nonoperative treatment for acute scaphoid fractures: a systematic review and meta-analysis of randomized controlled trials. J Trauma 2011; 71(4):1073–81.

68. Clay NR, Dias JJ, Costigan PS, et al. Need the thumb be immobilized in scaphoid fractures? A randomized prospective trial. J Bone Joint Surg Br 1991;73B:828–32.

69. Buijze GA, Goslings JC, Rhemrev SJ, et al. Cast immobilization with and without immobilization of the thumb for nondisplaced and minimally displaced scaphoid waist fractures: a multicenter, randomized, controlled trial. J Hand Surg Am 2014; 39(4):621–7.

70. Dias JJ, Wildin CJ, Bhowal B, et al. Should acute scaphoid fractures be fixed? A randomized controlled trial. J Bone Joint Surg Am 2005;87(10): 2160–8.

71. Dias JJ, Dhukaram V, Abhinav A, et al. Clinical and radiological outcome of cast immobilisation versus surgical treatment of acute scaphoid fractures at a mean follow-up of 93 months. J Bone Joint Surg Br 2008;90(7):899–905.

72. Saeden B, Tornkvist H, Ponzer S, et al. Fracture of the carpal scaphoid. A prospective, randomised 12-year follow-up comparing operative and conservative treatment. J Bone Joint Surg Br 2001;83(2): 230–4.

73. Miric D, Vuckovic C, Djordjevic Z. Radiographic signs of scaphoid union after bone grafting: the analysis of inter-observer agreement and intra-observer reproducibility. Srp Arh Celok Lek 2005; 133(3–4):142–5 [in Serbian].

74. Krimmer H, Schmitt R, Herbert T. Scaphoid fractures–diagnosis, classification and therapy. Unfallchirurg 2000;103(10):812–9.

75. Al-Ajmi TA, Al-Faryan KH, Al-Kanaan NF, et al. A systematic review and meta-analysis of randomized controlled trials comparing surgical versus conservative treatments for acute undisplaced or minimally-displaced scaphoid fractures. Clin Orthop Surg 2018;10:64–73.

76. Davis EN, Chung KC, Kotsis SV, et al. A cost/utility analysis of open reduction and internal fixation versus cast immobilization for acute nondisplaced mid-waist scaphoid fractures. Plast Reconstr Surg 2006;117(4):1223–35.

77. Ring D, Jupiter JB, Herndon JH. Acute fractures of the scaphoid. J Am Acad Orthop Surg 2000;8(4):225–31.

78. Andjelkovic SZ, Vuckovic CD, Lesic AR, et al. Fractures of the scaphoid, diagnosis and management– a review. Acta Chir Iugosl 2013;60(2):99–102.

79. Krimmer H. Management of acute fractures and nonunions of the proximal pole of the scaphoid. J Hand Surg 2002;27B(3):245–8.

80. Downing ND, Oni JA, Davis TR, et al. The relationship between proximal pole blood flow and the subjective assessment of increased density of the proximal pole in acute scaphoid fractures. J Hand Surg 2002;27A(3):402–8.

81. Trumble TE, Gilbert M, Murray LW, et al. Displaced scaphoid fractures treated with open reduction and internal fixation with a cannulated screw. J Bone Joint Surg Am 2000;82A(5):633–9.

82. Slade JF, Grauer JN, Mahoney JD. Arthroscopic reduction and percutaneous fixation of scaphoid fractures with a novel dorsal technique. Orthop Clin North Am 2001;32:247–61.

83. Slade JF, Gutow AP, Geissler WB. Percutaneous internal fixation of scaphoid fractures via an arthroscopically assisted dorsal approach. J Bone Joint Surg Am 2002;84A(suppl 2):21–36.

84. Dodds SD, Panjabi MM, Slade JF. Screw fixation of scaphoid fractures: a biomechanical assessment of screw length and screw augmentation. J Hand Surg Am 2006;31(3):405–13.

85. McCallister WV, Knight J, Kaliappan R, et al. Central placement of the screw in simulated fractures of the scaphoid waist: a biomechanical study. J Bone Joint Surg Am 2003;85(1):72–7.

86. Chan KW, McAdams TR. Central screw placement in percutaneous screw scaphoid fixation: a cadaveric comparison of proximal and distal techniques. J Hand Surg Am 2004;29(1):74–9.

87. Trumble TE, Clarke T, Kreder HJ. Non-union of the scaphoid. Treatment with cannulated screws compared with treatment with Herbert screws. J Bone Joint Surg Am 1996;78(12):1829–37.

88. Geurt SG, van Riet R, Meermans G, et al. Incidence of scaphotrapezial arthritis following volar percutaneous fixation of nondisplaced scaphoid waist fractures using a transtrapezial approach. J Hand Surg Am 2011;36(11):1753–8.

89. Kang KB, Kim HJ, Park JH, et al. Comparison of dorsal and volar percutaneous approaches in acute scaphoid fractures: a meta-analysis. PLoS One 2016;11(9):e0162779.

90. Slade JF, Jaskwhich D. Percutaneous fixation of scaphoid fractures. Hand Clin 2001;17:553–74.

91. Bain GI, Bennett JD, Richards RS, et al. Longitudinal computer tomography of the scaphoid: a new technique. Skeletal Radiol 1995;24:271–3.

92. Singh HP, Forward D, Davis TR, et al. Partial union of acute scaphoid fractures. J Hand Surg Br 2005;30(5):440–5.

93. Clementson M, Jorgsholm P, Besjakov J, et al. Union of scaphoid waist fractures assessed by CT scan. J Wrist Surg 2015;4(1):49–55.

94. Grewal R, Suh N, Macdermid JC. Use of computed tomography to predict union and time to union in acute scaphoid fractures treated nonoperatively. J Hand Surg Am 2013;38(5):872–7.

95. Eastley N, Singh H, Dias JJ, et al. Union rates after proximal scaphoid fractures; meta-analyses and review of available evidence. J Hand Surg Eur Vol 2013;38(8):888–97.

96. Brekke AC, Snoddy MC, Lee DH, et al. Biomechanical strength of the scaphoid partial union. J Wrist Surg 2018;7(5):399–403.

97. Riester JN, Baker BE, Mosher JF, et al. A review of scaphoid fracture healing in competitive athletes. Am J Sports Med 1985;13(3):159–61.

98. Halim A, Weiss AP. Return to play after hand and wrist fractures. Clin Sports Med 2016;35(4):597–608.

The Author's Technique for the Management of Unstable Scaphoid Nonunions
Tips and Tricks

Diego L. Fernandez, MD*

KEYWORDS

- Scaphoid nonunion • Interpositional bone grafting • Technique • Management

KEY POINTS

- This article presents the historical aspects, rationale, indications, planning, and execution of anterior interpositional bone grafting technique for unstable scaphoid nonunions.
- In the author's original technique, four points were considered: (1) the use of preoperative planning based on comparative anteroposterior radiographs in maximal ulnar deviation were used to calculate the resection zone, the size of the graft, and the scaphoid length; (2) a volar approach was used; (3) an iliac crest wedge-shaped corticocancellous graft was interposed; and (4) Kirschner wires were inserted for fixation.
- Contemporary refinements of the technique including a modification to treat nonunions with failed previous screw fixation with tricks and hints and results are shown.

INTRODUCTION

Scaphoid nonunions have a known natural history,[1,2] not all are symptomatic,[3] not all destabilize the carpus, but symptoms are accelerated by strenuous use of the hand. The two most important factors that affect obtaining bony union are the time elapsed between initial injury and treatment, and the presence of avascular necrosis of the proximal fragment.[4,5] These parameters, and the presence of periscaphoid degenerative changes, must be carefully evaluated because they represent major impediments to achieve a successful outcome with bone grafting techniques. Herbert[6–8] classified scaphoid nonunions in four types:

1. Fibrous union (without deformity)
2. Pseudarthrosis (early deformity)
3. Sclerotic pseudarthrosis (advanced deformity)
4. Avascular pseudarthrosis (fragmented proximal pole)

The currently accepted algorithm for the management scaphoid nonunion based on this classification is the following:

1. Fibrous nonunions (or delayed union): these are stable with absent deformity or collapse, have an excellent prognosis, should all be repaired, bone grafting is not necessary, and percutaneous screw fixation with arthroscopic or fluoroscopic control is the method of choice.[9]
2. Mobile nonunions: are unstable, have early collapse patterns (dorsal intercalated segmental instability [DISI]), a good prognosis, and require anterior wedge grafting and screw fixation to correct deformity. Compressed cancellous grafts with open or arthroscopic-assisted techniques may also be used.

Disclosure Statement: None.
University of Bern, Bern, Switzerland
* Chemin de la Côte du Bas 12, Cudrefin 1588, Switzerland.
E-mail address: diegof@bluewin.ch

Hand Clin 35 (2019) 271–279
https://doi.org/10.1016/j.hcl.2019.03.010

3. Sclerotic nonunions: are unstable, have moderate to marked collapse and early degenerative changes, ischemic proximal poles, and therefore carry a fair prognosis. A reconstruction trial is recommended according to age, occupation, and symptoms. Vascularized bone grafting may be indicated in this category if there is impaired perfusion of the proximal fragment.

4. Avascular nonunions: have nonreconstructable fragmented proximal poles. These have a poor prognosis, and therefore the proximal pole may be replaced by an osteochondral vascularized bone graft,[10] a costochondral graft,[11,12] or a prosthesis.[13] A salvage procedure may also be indicated.

In general terms, the categories of reconstruction of nonunited scaphoid are divided into:

1. An established nonunion without secondary degenerative changes within the wrist in which sound union of the scaphoid is the major goal

2. A scaphoid nonunion with early radioscaphoid degenerative changes in which union of the scaphoid has to be combined with an additional procedure, such as a radial styloidectomy[14]

3. A scaphoid nonunion with advanced degenerative wrist arthritis (scaphoid nonunion advanced collapse [SNAC] wrist III) for which only a salvage procedure, such as scaphoidectomy and four-corner fusion or proximal row carpectomy, is recommended

For the first category, the surgical considerations are based on the concept of stability, the location of the nonunion, and the presence or absence of osteonecrosis of the proximal fragment. Stable, nonunited scaphoid fractures in an anatomically acceptable position still profit from conventional inlay bone grafting.[5,15-20] The classic Matti-Russe[17-21] procedure is still a valid indication and is associated with high union rates, if the proximal fragment is well vascularized. Perhaps the only disadvantage is the long period of postoperative cast immobilization for at least 3 months.

The surgical management of the unstable, angulated, or displaced nonunions located at the scaphoid waist or distal third along with intact blood supply to the proximal pole is based on gaining more anatomic intrascaphoid angles and scaphoid length. This is best accomplished with an anteriorly placed interpositional wedge graft along with stable internal fixation.[6,22-27]

It has become clear from the data in several publications[1-3,7,28-30] that nonunited fractures of the scaphoid associated with displacement, deformity and shortening, and malunited fractures

have a higher incidence of associated osteoarthritis and impaired wrist function. In one study by Jiranek and associates,[31] more than 50% of patients treated for a scaphoid nonunion with a conventional inlay bone graft were found to have united with deformity. Although there was no significant subjective difference between those patients whose scaphoid healed anatomically compared with those with a malunion, there was a noteworthy difference in the functional results between these two groups. Furthermore Tsuyuguchi and associates[32] and others[22,30] also found a statistically significant correlation between improved wrist function and improved carpal alignment following anterior wedge-shaped grafting for an established scaphoid nonunion.

ASSESSMENT OF SCAPHOID NONUNION DEFORMITY

Unstable nonunions of the scaphoid exhibit the following deformity (based on the position of the distal fragment):

a. Flexion (humpback deformity)
b. Ulnar deviation (radial angulation)
c. Pronation (rotatory malalignment)
d. Shortening
e. Occasionally translation (step-offs)

With the advent of computed tomography (CT) and three-dimensional reconstruction, accurate imaging of normal scaphoid anatomy and deformity in nonunions and malunions became possible.

Scaphoid deformity and determination of the intrascaphoid angles[33] has been thoroughly analyzed with three-spiral tomography, CT scans,[34,35] and three-dimensional reconstruction.[36] Bain and colleagues[37] refined the lateral intrascaphoid angle measurement using longitudinal CT scans[34] and described the dorsal scaphoid angle and the height-to-length ratio as further measurement techniques.

It was concluded that fractures distal to the apex of the dorsal ridge usually develop a palmar type of late deformity (flexion and overhang of the distal fragment), whereas fractures of the proximal third develop a dorsal type of late deformity with dorsal "slipping" of the distal fragment without carpal malalignment.[36,38] The defect following reduction of the scaphoid fragments to match the contralateral side was studied by Oka and colleagues.[39] The palmar type of deformity (waist) resulted in larger triangular defects, whereas proximal nonunions exhibited a flat crescent-like smaller defect.

Schweizer and colleagues[40] described a dorsal or dorsoradial overlapping of the fragments following virtual reduction. Failure to remove excess bone dorsally would shift the center of rotation dorsally, create a larger gap, and therefore result in an overcorrection of scaphoid length and limited radial deviation. Resection of dorsal new bone or "callus" formation was, however, not recommended to prevent damage to the dorsal ridge nourishing vessels.

ANTERIOR WEDGE GRAFTING TECHNIQUE

Anterior interpositional bone grafting technique is my current method of choice for unstable, deformed, and angulated nonunions located at the waist or at the distal third of the carpal scaphoid with a viable proximal fragment. Restoration of normal scaphoid length through distraction of the nonunion restores the "strut" function of the radial column of the carpus, which in turn controls the initial carpal collapse and the associated dorsal lunate rotation.[24]

Preoperative Planning

The only component of the deformity that can be approximately calculated with plain radiographs is the scaphoid length using maximally ulnar deviated anteroposterior views of both wrists. The amount of resection and size of the graft needed in millimeters are calculated preoperatively by carefully tracing the radiographic findings of the affected and normal scaphoids in the frontal plane (**Fig. 1**B).[24] Using CT scan cuts in the long axis of the scaphoid[34] the anteroposterior and lateral intrascaphoid angles, the dorsal cortical angle, and the height-to-length ratio[37] can be measured. The amount of correction is given by the difference of the values of the deformed and the contralateral normal scaphoid. Accordingly Kirschner wires can be inserted in the scaphoid fragments subtending the correction angles in nonunions and malunions (**Fig. 2**B).[41,42] If three-dimensional reconstruction is used, the size and form of the defect to be grafted is given by the virtual correction.

Historical Evolution of the Technique

In the early 1970s, Segmüller[43] pointed out that shortening of the scaphoid was detrimental for normal carpal kinematics and proposed a technique of interpositional or "sandwich" grafting through a dorsal approach. Following resection of the sclerotic edges, a rectangular-shaped "compression-resistant" corticocancellous iliac graft was inserted and scaphoid length was restored with a spreader clamp. The author stressed the need for accurate screw placement mainly because, in most scaphoid nonunions, the

plane of the nonunion is not perpendicular to the long axis of the scaphoid. Lag screw fixation was strongly advocated to neutralize micromotion, enhance undisturbed healing, and permit a less cumbersome postoperative management, reducing the duration of wrist immobilization in a cast.

Later in the same decade, Fisk[44–46] recognized the association of dorsal carpal instability patterns with the humpback or flexion deformity of the scaphoid, stating that in the presence of carpal instability the proximal fragment of the scaphoid generally tilts backward with the lunate and the distal fragment forward with the capitate. This opens up the fracture site in the dorsal aspect and is one cause for nonunion. Resorption of the anterior margins of the fracture takes place so that the scaphoid collapses in length and becomes "hump-backed," the distal and proximal poles pointing forward.

In Fisk's technique,[45] the scaphoid is approached through a radial incision with styloidectomy. After curetting out the fibrous tissue and adding multiple drill holes to the sclerotic surfaces, the DISI deformity is corrected manually with palmar translation of the distal carpus. This maneuver opens the scaphoid gap anterolaterally. A wedge of appropriate size is cut from the resected radial styloid and fitted into the defect. Fisk did not consider internal fixation necessary and stated that: "...when the traction is released, the resilience of the soft tissues holds the graft firmly into position..." Postoperatively, the wrist was immobilized for 2 to 3 months.

In 1982, the author modified the Fisk procedure to treat scaphoid nonunions associated with carpal instability, and the early results obtained with this technique were reported in 1984.[24] The author's goal was to try to restore the anatomic shape and length of the scaphoid based on the use of comparative radiographs of the noninjured wrist. A careful preoperative plan using tracing paper enabled the authors to measure the length of both scaphoids and to calculate in millimeters the size and shape of the iliac crest graft to fit the defect after resection of the nonunion (**Fig. 1**A, C; see **Fig. 1**B). The scapholunate angle was used to assess the correction of the associated DISI pattern of carpal instability. Additional modifications included the use of a palmar approach and internal fixation with two or three Kirschner wires.

Current Technique

An extended volar Russe approach is used. The capsule is incised in line with the skin incision.

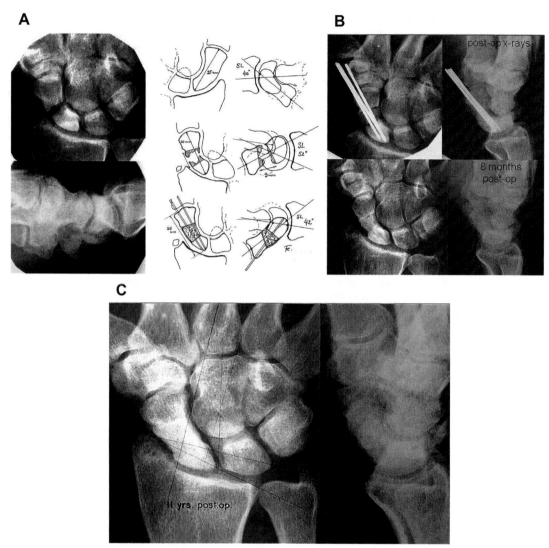

Fig. 1. (*A*) Unstable scaphoid waist nonunion following closed reduction and casting of a trans-scapho perilunar dislocation. Notice sclerosis of the proximal fragment and the dorsally rotated lunate. The amount of resection, size of the graft, and restoration of scaphoid length are planned with tracings of the opposite wrist. (*B, Top*) Roentgenograms following interpositional bone grafting. Notice restoration of the scaphoid anatomy and correction of the DISI deformity. (*B, Bottom*) Radiographic result at 8 months showing undisturbed bony healing, a well-remodeled graft, and good carpal alignment. (*C*) At 11 years late follow-up, radiographs reveal a well-maintained carpal alignment and absence of degenerative changes. (*From* Fernandez DL. A technique for anterior wedge-shaped grafts for scaphoid nonunions with carpal instability. J Hand Surg 1984;9(5):733–7; with permission.)

The capsular flaps that contain the strong radio-scaphocapite ligament are held on both sides with stay sutures to facilitate anatomic closure. Sclerotic or irregular borders of the nonunion site are then resected with a small oscillating saw to offer a perfect surface contact between the graft and the scaphoid fragments. Additional cystic defects are curetted out and filled with small cancellous bone chips. The flexion deformity and shortening of the scaphoid are corrected by distracting the osteotomized surfaces on the palmar radial aspect with a small spreader clamp, or simply by hyperextending the wrist over a rolled towel. The bone defect should correspond to the dimensions calculated preoperatively. As this is done, the surgical assistant simultaneously corrects the dorsal rotation of the lunate by pushing the palmar pole toward the radius with a fine bone spike or by using a Kirschner wire as a joystick inserted through the palmar pole of the lunate to control rotation. The corticocancellous graft is obtained from the iliac crest and shaped

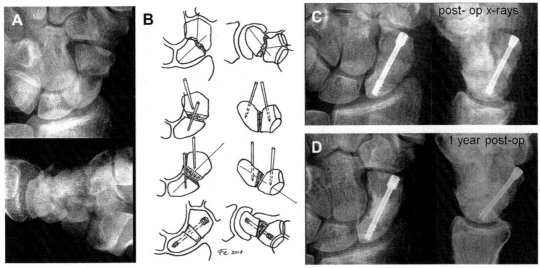

Fig. 2. (*A*) Unstable cystic nonunion. Notice shortening, "ad latus" translation of the distal fragment, flexion deformity in the sagittal plane, and DISI malalignment. (*B*) The Kirschner wires subtend the angles of deformity in the horizontal plane (pronation of the distal fragment) and flexion in the sagittal plane. After resection of the nonunion edges, the deformity is corrected extending and supinating the distal fragment until both Kirschner wires are parallel to each other in both planes. After placing the graft, a cannulated headless screw is inserted. Roentgenograms immediately after surgery (*C*) and at 1 year (*D*). Image shows adequate restoration of the scaphoid length and correction of angular deformity and normal carpal alignment. ([*B*] *Adapted from* Fernandez DL, Martin CJ, Gonzalez del Pino J. Scaphoid malunion: the significance of rotational malalignment. The Journal of Hand Surgery: British & European Volume 1998;23(6):773; with permission.)

according to the preoperative plan and the intraoperative dimensions of the bone defect and is inserted with the cortical part of the graft being oriented palmarly.

Another way to correct the humpback deformity is to use 1.2-mm Kirschner wires inserted in each fragment of the scaphoid, allowing one to open the nonunion site and correct the flexion deformity in the sagittal plane, and the pronation of the distal fragment in the horizontal plane. In order not to interfere with the central screw track for final fixation, the distal wire is placed ulnar and the proximal wire radial to the central long axis of the scaphoid.[41] These wires can be used as joysticks and after completing reduction the Kirschner wires should be parallel to each other (**Fig. 2**).

If computer-assisted three-dimensional reconstruction is used, patient-specific guides are three-dimensional printed and used to insert two Kirschner wires in each fragment subtending the angular correction in all three planes. Following reduction, a second guide to hold the Kirschner wires parallel is applied and maintained during grafting and screw insertion.[47]

Finally, a headless cannulated compression screw is inserted for fixation of the scaphoid. If access to the central axis of the scaphoid is difficult, the anterior border of the trapezium

is removed to facilitate the correct point of entry of the guidewire. Alternatively, the transtrapezoidal guidewire insertion to ensure optimal screw placement is strongly recommended.[48] The latter subtends an angle of 45° with the long axis of the forearm in the frontal and sagittal planes. Usually the headless screw should be 4 mm shorter than the length of the guidewire within the scaphoid. If cannulated systems are not available, temporary fixation of both scaphoid fragments and the graft with a separate Kirschner wire is strongly recommended to avoid displacement of the interposed graft during drilling and tapping.

If a long-standing DISI deformity is present with a radiolunate angle greater than 20°, usually additional pinning of the lunate to the radius for 6 to 8 weeks is advisable to prevent recurrence of carpal malalignment.[49] Through the volar approach, lunate derotation from the extended to a neutral position (radiolunate angle 0°) is performed either by using a 1.6-mm Kirschner wire inserted into the lunate through the palmar pole as a joystick, or by simply flexing the wrist as suggested by Linscheid.[49,50] Occasionally radiocarpal adhesions in the radiolunate joint have to be released with a dissector through the volar approach. Having verified correct lunate rotation, a 1.2-mm Kirschner wire is driven through the distal radius across the radiocarpal joint into the body of the lunate.

Careful closure of the palmar capsule with fine nonresorbable sutures completes the operation, and a radial plaster splint that includes the thumb is applied postoperatively for 2 weeks.

Postoperative Management

Wrist immobilization is discontinued at 2 weeks after the operation except in those cases in which Kirschner wire fixation of the lunate across the radius is needed for the first 8 weeks. Should postoperative pain persist at 2 weeks, a removable plastic splint or wrist brace may be used for another 2 to 4 weeks. The patient is encouraged to use the hand for activities of daily living. However, heavy manual work and strenuous sport activities are forbidden until 8 weeks after surgery. At this time, the first radiographs are taken. The author's criteria to establish healing are:

1. The absence of pain
2. The radiographic evidence of bridging bony trabeculae on both sides of the interposed graft
3. Disappearance of the osteotomy lines in conventional radiographs
4. No signs of screw loosening

If there is any doubt regarding radiographic healing, CT scans may be used to confirm bony union.

ILIAC PEG AND "ARC DE TRIOMPHE GRAFT" TECHNIQUE

This personal technique is indicated for scaphoid nonunions with failed screw fixation and a viable proximal pole. Usually the loose screw produces an additional longitudinal bone defect in the proximal and distal fragments. For these cases, after having checked the vascularity of the proximal pole (at least two bleeding points) an iliac peg corticocancellous strut placed in the screw channel is combined with an anterior wedge graft. To fit over the longitudinal peg a notch is created in the center of the wedge by removing enough cancellous bone with a fine rongeur. Because it is shaped like an arch the author calls it "arc de triomphe" graft (**Fig. 3**A–D).

A volar extended Russe approach is used. The loose screw is removed and scar tissue is curetted out of the screw channel. Resection of the nonunion site is carried out with a mini oscillating saw. To facilitate the placement of the peg graft I recommend to remove the bone directly over the screw channel on the distal fragment volarly.

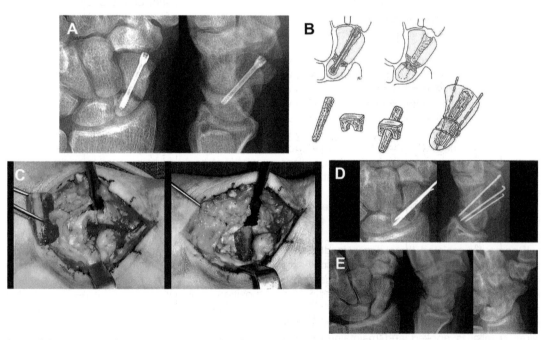

Fig. 3. (*A*) Nonunion of the proximal pole after failed screw fixation. Notice osteolytic zone around the screw channel. (*B, Top*) Following resection of the nonunion site and curettage of the screw channel, the bone directly over the screw channel on the distal fragment is removed to facilitate insertion of the peg graft in the proximal pole. (*B, Bottom*) Schematic representation of the assembled graft and its placement. The nonunion is stabilized with two axial Kirschner wires. (*C*) Intraoperative photographs of both grafts in place. (*D*) Immediate postoperative radiographs that (*E*) at l6 months reveal a healed scaphoid with solid osseous integration of the grafts.

Therefore, the peg is an inlay graft distally and intramedullary in the proximal fragment. If attempts are done to force the peg from distal to proximal in the old screw channel more than often the peg may fracture. However, if it goes in loosely it could be done, but most probably the graft will not have a snug fit.

Before inserting the interpositional graft on top of the peg be sure and fill all spaces with free cancellous bone chips. Next, the wedge graft is fitted and impacted being careful not to damage the underlying peg graft. Internal fixation is performed with two or three 1.25-mm Kirschner wires inserted from distal to proximal. Screw fixation is contraindicated because there is little bone left in the proximal fragment to guarantee solid screw purchase.

Postoperatively a dorsoradial splint is applied for 2 weeks. Following suture removal, a forearm cast including the base of the thumb is applied for 8 weeks.

Scaphoid views and CT scans are done between 8 and 10 weeks following surgery. If bridging trabeculae are confirmed on both sides of the interposed graft immobilization is discontinued and wrist rehabilitation begun. More than often the Kirschner wire ends in the thenar region may disturb the patient and need to be removed under local anesthesia.

Pearls and Pitfalls of the Technique

Pearls

1. Be sure the proximal fragment has adequate vascularity
2. Careful manual shaping of both grafts to adapt into the bone defect is mandatory
3. Remove the volar bone over the distal screw channel to facilitate insertion and make sure there is a snug fit to the axial peg graft

Pitfalls

1. Fracture of the peg graft caused by forceful insertion in the old screw channel
2. Failure to obtain adequate Kirschner wire placement in the proximal fragment
3. Early migration of Kirschner wire leading to skin irritation
4. Cast immobilization shorter than 8 weeks

RESULTS

Several publications have reported favorable results with interpositional anterior bone grafting techniques.[6,41,51,52] Watanabe[53] showed good restoration of carpal alignment according to the preoperative plan in 38 patients comparing the intrascaphoid angles, scaphoid length, and radiolunate and scapholunate angles preoperatively and postoperatively and with the contralateral side.

In a systematic review on the graft choice for unstable scaphoid nonunions[54] analyzing 604 patients in 23 studies it could be shown that cancellous bone graft provides the shortest interval to union, whereas corticocancellous grafts are associated with consistent deformity correction and superior Mayo Wrist Scores. This is most probably because corticocancellous grafts have a higher compression resistance than cancellous grafts. Tambe and colleagues[55] reported that the union rate of scaphoid nonunions treated with iliac bone or distal radius grafts was comparable, although the quality of the iliac bone is superior.

The author's results[22,27] have shown that reestablishment of normal scaphoid anatomy and resolution of the scaphoid nonunion advanced collapse deformity. We reported 40 scaphoid nonunions treated with interpositional volar wedge grafting, of which 24 were located at the waist, 12 in the proximal pole, two in the proximal third, and two in the distal pole. The average follow-up was 5.7 years (range, 2–11.9 years). The average healing rate was 89%. There were five persistent nonunions. One waist nonunion failed to heal and the other four were associated with avascularity of the proximal pole. Thirty-eight out of 40 patients returned to their previous occupation and the overall patient satisfaction was 92%. The overall ratings according to the Mayo Clinic Wrist Score were 15 excellent, 13 good, five fair, and seven poor. The overall radiographic assessment showed that carpal alignment was restored and maintained, and that mild degenerative changes were present in 25% of the patients. However, even in those patients with mild preoperative signs of arthrosis, there was no radiographic progression of degenerative changes in healed nonunions at late follow-up. It was concluded that restoration of scaphoid length and correction of angular deformity stopped further carpal collapse therefore postponing or diminishing the progression of degenerative wrist disease.

REFERENCES

1. Ruby LK, Stinson J, Belsky MR. The natural history of scaphoid non-union: a review of fifty-five cases. J Bone Joint Surg Am 1985;67A:428–32.
2. Mack GR, Bosse MJ, Gelberman RH, et al. The natural history of scaphoid non-union. J Bone Joint Surg Am 1984;66A:504–9.

3. Lindström G, Nyström A. Natural history of scaphoid non-union with special reference to "asymptomatic" cases. J Hand Surg 1992;17B:697–700.

4. Schuind F, Haentjens P, Van Innis F, et al. Prognostic factors in the treatment of carpal scaphoid non-unions. J Hand Surg 1999;24A:761–76.

5. Green DP. The effect of avascular necrosis on Russe bone grafting for scaphoid nonunion. J Hand Surg 1985;10A:597–605.

6. Herbert TJ, Fisher WE. Management of the fractured scaphoid using a new bone screw. J Bone Joint Surg Am 1984;66B:114–23.

7. Herbert TJ. The fractured scaphoid. St Louis (MO): Quality Medical Publishing; 1990.

8. Filan SL, Herbert TJ. Herbert screw fixation of scaphoid fractures. J Bone Joint Surg Am 1996; 78B:519–29.

9. Slade JF, Geissler WB, Gutow AP, et al. Percutaneous internal fixation of selected scaphoid non-unions with an arthroscopically assisted dorsal approach. J Bone Joint Surg Am 2003;85A(Supp. 4):20–32.

10. Burger HK, Windhofer C, Gaggl AJ, et al. Vascularized medial femoral trochlea osteocartilaginous flap reconstruction of proximal pole scaphoid non-unions. J Hand Surg Am 2013;38(4):690–700.

11. Sandow MJ. Costo-osteochondral grafts in the wrist. Tech Hand Up Extrem Surg 2001;5(3):165–72.

12. Yao J, Read B, Hentz VR. The fragmented proximal pole scaphoid nonunion treated with rib autograft: case series and review of the literature. J Hand Surg Am 2013;38(11):2188–92.

13. Pequinot JP, Lussiez B, Allieu Y. An adaptative proximal scaphoid implant. Chir Main 2000;19(5): 276–85.

14. Mazet R Jr, Hohl M. Radial styloidectomy and styloidectomy plus bone graft in the treatment of old ununited carpal scaphoid fractures. Ann Surg 1960; 152:296–302.

15. Cooney WP, Dobyns JH, Linscheid RL. Fractures of the scaphoid: a rational approach to management. Clin Orthop 1980;(149):90–7.

16. Kleinert JM, Zenni EJ Jr. Nonunion of the scaphoid: review of literature and current treatment. Orthop Rev 1984;13:125–41.

17. Russe O. Fracture of the carpal navicular: diagnosis, non-operative treatment, and operative treatment. J Bone Joint Surg Am 1960;42A:759–68.

18. Andrews J, Miller G, Haddad R. Treatment of scaphoid nonunion by volar inlay distal radius bone graft. J Hand Surg 1985;10B:214–6.

19. Warren-Smith CD, Barton NJ. Non-union of the scaphoid: Russe graft vs. Herbert screw. J Hand Surg 1988;13B:83–6.

20. Schneider LH, Aulicino P. Nonunion of the carpal scaphoid: the Russe procedure. J Trauma 1982;22: 315–9.

21. Matti H. Über die Behandlung der Navicularefraktur und der Refractura patellae durch Plombierung mit Spongiosa. Zentralbl Chir 1937;64:2353–9.

22. Fernandez DL. Anterior bone grafting and conventional lag screw fixation to treat scaphoid non-unions. J Hand Surg 1990;15A:140–7.

23. Stark HH, Rickard TA, Zemel NP, et al. Treatment of ununited fractures of the scaphoid by iliac bone grafts and Kirschner-wire fixation. J Bone Joint Surg Am 1988;70A:982–91.

24. Fernandez DL. A technique for anterior wedge-shaped grafts for scaphoid nonunions with carpal instability. J Hand Surg 1984;9A:733–7.

25. Cooney WP, Linscheid RL, Dobyns JH, et al. Scaphoid nonunion: role of anterior interpositional bone grafts. J Hand Surg 1988;13A:635–50.

26. Fernandez DL, Eggli S. Scaphoid nonunion and malunion: how to correct deformity. Hand Clin 2001;17-4:631–46.

27. Eggli S, Fernandez DL, Beck TH. Unstable scaphoid non-union: a medium-term study of anterior wedge grafting procedures. J Hand Surg 2002;27B:36–41.

28. Kaneshiro SA, Failla JM, Tashman S. Scaphoid fracture displacement with forearm rotation in a short-arm thumb spica cast. J Hand Surg 1999;24A: 984–91.

29. Nakamura R, Imaeda T, Tsuge S, et al. Scaphoid non-union with D.I.S.I. deformity. A survey of clinical cases with special reference to ligamentous injury. J Hand Surg 1991;16A:156–61.

30. Steiger R, Sennwald G. Late results of operated scaphoid pseudarthroses. Handchir Mikrochir Plast Chir 1990;22:152–5.

31. Jiranek WA, Ruby LK, Millender LB, et al. Long-term results after Russe bone-grafting: the effect of malunion of the scaphoid. J Bone Joint Surg Am 1992; 74A:1217–28.

32. Tsuyuguchi Y, Murase T, Hidaka N, et al. Anterior wedge-shaped bone graft for old scaphoid fractures or non-unions. J Hand Surg 1995;20B:194–200.

33. Amadio PC, Berquist TH, Smith DK, et al. Scaphoid malunion. J Hand Surg 1989;14A:679–87.

34. Sanders WE. Evaluation of the humpback scaphoid by computed tomography in the longitudinal axial plane of the scaphoid. J Hand Surg 1988;13A: 182–7.

35. Belsole RJ, Hilbelink DR, Llewellyn JA, et al. Computed analysis of the pathomechanics of scaphoid waist nonunions. J Hand Surg 1991;16A: 899–906.

36. Nakamura R, Imaeda T, Horii E, et al. Analysis of scaphoid fracture displacement by three-dimensional computed tomography. J Hand Surg 1991;16A:485–92.

37. Bain GI, Bennett JD, MacDermid JC, et al. Measurement of the scaphoid humpback deformity using longitudinal computed tomography: intra and

interobserver variability using various measurement techniques. J Hand Surg 1998;23A:76–81.

38. Moritomo H, Viegas SF, Elder KW, et al. Scaphoid nonunions: a 3-dimensional analysis of patterns of deformity. J Hand Surg 2000;25A:520–8.

39. Oka K, Murase T, Moritomo H, et al. Patterns of bone defect in scaphoid nonunion: a 3-dimensional and quantitative analysis. J Hand Surg 2005;30A:359–65.

40. Schweizer A, Fürnstahl PH, Nagy L. Three-dimensional computed tomographic analysis of 11 scaphoid waist nonunions. J Hand Surg 2012;37A:1151–8.

41. Bindra R, Bednar M, Light T. Volar wedge grafting for scaphoid non-union with collapse. J Hand Surg 2008;33A:974–9.

42. Fernandez DL, Martin CL, Gonzalez del Pino J. Scaphoid malunion: the significance of rotational malalignment. J Hand Surg 1998;23B:771–5.

43. Segmüller G. Operative stabilisierung am handskelett. Bern (Switzerland): Hans Huber Verlag; 1973.

44. Fisk GR. Carpal instability and the fractured scaphoid. Ann R Coll Surg Engl 1970;46:63–76.

45. Fisk GR. Operative orthopaedics part III. Butterworth (Malaysia): George Bentley; 1979.

46. Fisk GR. An overview of injuries of the wrist. Clin Orthop 1980;149:137–44.

47. Schweizer A, Mauler F, Vlachopoulos L, et al. Computer-assisted 3dimensional reconstructions of scaphoid fractures and nonunions with and without the use of patient-specific guides: early clinical outcomes and postoperative assessments of reconstruction accuracy. J Hand Surg Am 2016;41:59–69.

48. Meermans G, van Gabbeck F, Braem MJ, et al. Comparison of two percutaneous volar approaches for screw fixation of scaphoid waist fractures: radiographic and biomechanical study of an osteotomy simulated model. J Bone Joint Surg Am 2014;96(16):1369–76.

49. Linscheid RL, Dobyns JB, Cooney WP. Volar wedge grafting of the carpal scaphoid in non-union associated with dorsal instability patterns. J Bone Joint Surg Am 1982;64B:632–3.

50. Tomaino MM, King J, Pizillo M. Correction of lunate malalignment when bone grafting scaphoid nonunion with humpback deformity: rationale and results of a technique revisited. J Hand Surg 2000;25A:322–9.

51. Rajagopalan BM, Squire DS, Samuels LO. Results of Herbert-screw fixation with bone grafting for the treatment of nonunion of the scaphoid. J Bone Joint Surg Am 1999;81A:48–51.

52. Huang YC, Liu Y, Chen TH. Long-term results of scaphoid non-union treated by intercalated bone grafting and Herbert's screw fixation: a study of 49 patients for at least five years. Int Orthop 2009;33:1295–300.

53. Watanabe K. Analysis of carpal malalignment caused by scaphoid nonunion and evaluation of corrective bone graft on carpal alignment. J Hand Surg 2011;36A:10–6.

54. Sayegh ET, Strauch RJ. Graft choice in the management of unstable scaphoid nonunion: a systemic review. J Hand Surg 2014;39A:1500–6.

55. Tambe AD, Cutler L, Murali SR, et al. In scaphoid nonunion, does the source of graft affect outcome? Iliac crest versus distal end of radius bone graft. J Hand Surg 2006;31B:47–51.

The Authors' Technique for Volar Plating of Scaphoid Nonunion

Feiran Wu, MA, MB BChir (Cantab), FRCS (Tr & Orth),
Chye Yew Ng, FRCS (Tr & Orth), DipHandSurg (Br & Eur),
Mike Hayton, FRCS (Tr & Orth), FFSEM (UK)*

KEYWORDS

- Scaphoid • Nonunion • Volar plate • DISI • Humpback deformity • Fracture fixation

KEY POINTS

- The optimal management of scaphoid nonunions remains challenging.
- Salvage procedures such as proximal row carpectomy or scaphoid excision with four-corner arthrodesis can lead to reduced range of wrist motion and grip strength.
- Scaphoid plates provide considerably more buttress support than intramedullary headless screws.
- A volar approach also allows relatively straightforward correction of any fracture deformity, placement of bone graft, and internal plate fixation.
- Screw fixation in variable trajectories through the plate can control the angle and rotation of the fracture fragments and offer torsional rigidity, making this a useful tool in the reduction of fractures with significant humpback deformities.

INTRODUCTION

The optimal management of complex scaphoid fractures and scaphoid nonunions remains challenging. The current gold standard for scaphoid fracture fixation remains a headless compression screw, which provides structural support by compressing the proximal and distal fracture fragments.[1] It is also thought to prevent bending through a 3-point fixation mechanism within the cancellous bone of the scaphoid. The proximal and distal points of purchase are achieved by the capture of the screw threads in the proximal and distal poles. The third point occurs within the waist of the scaphoid and therefore requires little to no bone loss to provide a stable construct.

Despite optimal treatment, some acute scaphoid fractures do not heal. Risk factors for nonunion include delays in diagnosis, interfragmentary instability, and proximal location of the fracture with an increasingly poor retrograde vascular supply.[2] Unstable volar waist fractures are predisposed to fracture collapse and nonunion, because the edges of the proximal and distal pole fragments abut each other and after repeated cycles of loading, experience progressive erosion and bone loss. This causes the fracture to collapse into a humpback deformity and the remainder of the carpal bones develops a dorsal intercalated segment instability pattern.[3] In fractures with significant bone loss, screw fixation may be unable to maintain fragmentary stability due to the loss of the 3-point fixation

---

Disclosure Statement: M. Hayton is a paid member of the Medartis scaphoid plate development group but receives no royalties from the implant. This research received no specific grant from any funding agency in the public, commercial, or not-for-profit sectors.
Upper Limb Unit, Wrightington Hospital, Hall Lane, Appley Bridge, Wrightington, Wigan WN6 9EP, UK
* Corresponding author.
E-mail address: mikehayton@gmail.com

Hand Clin 35 (2019) 281–286
https://doi.org/10.1016/j.hcl.2019.03.009

mechanism, which can then progress to nonunion.[4,5]

Complex scaphoid nonunions have been described for those with failure of prior fixation, avascular necrosis at the proximal pole, and bone loss with cystic degeneration at the fracture site.[6–8] When facing these scenarios, salvage procedures in the form of proximal row carpectomy or scaphoid excision with 4-corner arthrodesis have been performed.[9] Although reliable in providing pain relief, both techniques can lead to reduced range of wrist motion and grip strength.[9] The establishment of newer techniques such as rigid plate fixation has enabled the surgery of scaphoid nonunions to be more predictable, which may reduce the morbidity associated with salvage procedures when successful.

Plate fixation of scaphoid fractures was first described by Ender in 1977 for the treatment of scaphoid fractures with significant volar bone loss and nonunion, who introduced a plate that was hooked on the proximal scaphoid fragment and fixed to the distal fragment of the scaphoid with a screw.[10] It was partly intraarticular, which often necessitated removal due to cartilage irritation on the radius.[11] Other described techniques of using plate fixation to treat scaphoid fractures include AO buttress plates[12] and dorsal locked mini-plates,[13] both of which demonstrated high union rates.

More recently, a volar extraarticular scaphoid plate has been introduced (Trilock 1.5, Medartis AG, Switzerland). This precontoured volar plate has several advantages over other small modular hand plates:

- Scaphoid morphology replicated.
- 0.8 mm low profile to reduce impingement.
- Locking and nonlocking screw options through each hole.
- Rigid radial and ulnar columns to improve rigidity particularly in cases requiring cancellous bone grafting.

Such a plate cannot achieve compression like a headless compression screw, but can provide considerably more buttress support and rigidity, particularly in the presence of bone loss. Screw fixation in variable trajectories through the plate can also theoretically control the angle and rotation of the proximal and distal fracture fragments and offer additional torsional rigidity, making this a useful tool in the reduction of fractures with significant humpback or flexion deformities.[14] Biomechanically, locked plates convert shear stress to compressive stress at the screw–bone interface, improving fixation because bone has much higher resistance to compressive than shear stress.[15]

Therefore, as scaphoid fractures tend to collapse in a predictable apex-dorsal humpback mechanism, such a contoured locked volar scaphoid plate provides the perfect mechanical construct that meets the anatomic and biomechanical requirements of these fractures.[5]

INDICATIONS

The indications for plating scaphoid fractures are evolving. Our criteria for plating of scaphoid fractures using a volar precontoured extraarticular plate include (1) acute unstable oblique fractures of the waist; (2) acute waist fractures with significant comminution or bone loss; (3) scaphoid nonunions with bone loss and/or a humpback deformity; and (4) complex scaphoid nonunions with central cavitation following failure of primary fixation using a headless screw. This plate is not suitable for small proximal pole nonunions.

TECHNIQUE
Surgical Approach

Patients are positioned supine with the injured hand extended on an arm table. Either general and/or regional anesthesia is used. An above elbow tourniquet is inflated and intraoperative fluoroscopy is essential. A volar nerve-sparing approach is used as described by Hagert and colleagues[16] for adequate exposure and visualization of the scaphoid (**Fig. 1**). A radiovolar skin incision is made centered over the flexor carpi radialis (FCR) tendon starting 4 cm proximal to the proximal wrist crease and curving radially to the scaphoid tubercle distal to the wrist crease. The superficial forearm fascia is incised longitudinally, the FCR sheath opened, and the tendon retracted ulnarward. The superficial palmar branch of the radial artery is identified and ligated. The deep forearm fascia is incised at the level at which it inserts into the lateral edge of the distal radius, just palmar to the brachioradialis tendon insertion and extended up to the tip of the radial styloid. The pronator quadratus is elevated subperiosteally from the distal radius, exposing the volar wrist capsule and radiocarpal ligaments. To easily define the oblique orientation of the extrinsic ligaments, the wrist can be radially and ulnarly deviated several times. The tip of the radial styloid is then identified and an oblique incision is made starting at the styloid and aiming toward the capitate, splitting the extrinsic ligaments parallel with their fibers. The scaphoid can now be seen at the base of this initial incision. The next incision involves releasing the radioscaphocapitate ligament

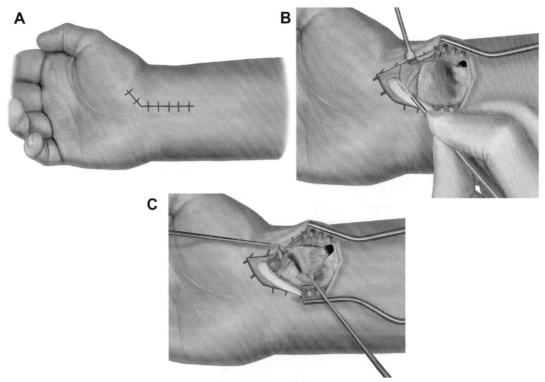

Fig. 1. (*A*) Radiovolar skin incision centered over the FCR tendon. (*B*) The incision through the capsule dividing the extrinsic ligaments. (*C*) The capsular flaps are elevated to expose the scaphoid. FCR, flexor carpi radialis. (*Courtesy of* M. Hayton, FRCS (Tr & Orth) FFSEM (UK), Wrightington, UK.)

off the distal edge of the radius in an ulnar direction. The final incision involves releasing the distal radial insertion of the radioscaphoid ligament off the scaphoid tubercle to allow retraction of the ligament in a radial direction.

This approach has the advantage of being ligament splitting in nature, allowing rapid healing of the obliquely orientated extrinsic ligaments. Additional benefit, particularly in the context of the scaphoid plate, is that it provides a wide exposure of the volar scaphoid surface that allows accurate fracture reduction and plate positioning, while preserving the anterior interosseous nerve innervation of the radial wrist ligaments.[16]

Bone Grafting

Autologous bone graft is used in acute fractures with significant bone loss and all nonunions. The pronator quadratus is released off the radial metaphysis for bone graft harvest. A 1.1 mm drill is used on the volar metaphyseal cortex to mark the corners of a square before an osteotome is used on 3 sides to elevate a cortical flap. Cancellous graft is harvested using a curette, and the cortical flap is replaced at the end of harvesting. The authors

do not believe vascularized graft is necessary using this technique, because the mechanical stability provided by the buttress plate offers an excellent biological environment for bone healing. However, a pedicled volar artery vascularized bone graft can be harvested using the same approach.

Scaphoid Preparation

The scaphoid nonunion requires meticulous preparation and removal of fibrous tissue and sclerotic bone at the pseudarthrosis site using a curette or circular burr at low speed under adequate irrigation (**Fig. 2**A). The opposing edges of the nonunion are further prepared with several Kirschner wire (K-wire) holes to increase the surface area at the nonunion surfaces. The fracture fragments are then brought into the anatomic position under fluoroscopy and stabilized with a 1.1 mm K-wire in an antegrade or retrograde direction depending on the fracture configuration (**Fig. 2**B). If necessary, the lunate is also reduced and held temporarily with a 1.1 mm K-wire inserted through the dorsal distal radius. In cases requiring autologous bone graft, the harvested bone is then impacted into the defect.

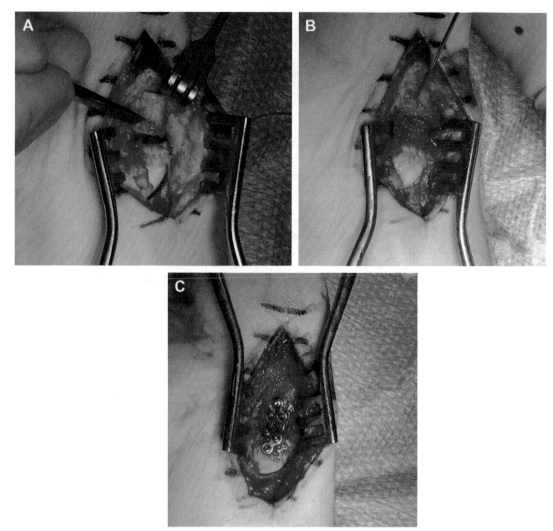

Fig. 2. (*A*) Fibrous tissue and sclerotic bone is cleared at the pseudarthrosis site. (*B*) The bone graft is positioned at the fracture site. (*C*) The precontoured volar plate is positioned onto the scaphoid.

Plate Position

It is important to ensure satisfactory placement of the plate onto the scaphoid (**Fig. 2**C). The Trilock 1.5 plate is designed to sit on the volar aspect of this bone and should appear centered on anteroposterior fluoroscopy. The plate position is confirmed by intraoperative fluoroscopy, and an initial nonlocking screw is placed in the proximal fracture fragment and tightened to bring the plate flush to the bone. The wrist is gently flexed to ensure the plate does not impinge on the volar rim of the radius and the remaining holes are then filled with locking screws. All screws have the added advantage of allowing 15° of variable angle for optimum purchase and to avoid joint penetration distally and proximally. Ideally all screw holes should be used, but nonsecured holes

remaining in the middle of the plate are not detrimental to the final implant construct.[5]

The proximal to distal positioning of the plate on the scaphoid can be challenging in more proximal fractures. Excessive proximal positioning of the plate onto the proximal pole can lead to plate impingement on volar flexion of the wrist at the radioscaphoid articulation, typically when the wrist flexes beyond 60°. In these situations, the most proximal hole can be clipped off the plate, although this may reduce its buttressing effect and construct stability as the working length is shortened as a result. It is not unreasonable to maintain fixation with a potentially impinging screw and remove a small area of the volar radial rim that would impinge in flexion rather than compromise fixation. If symptomatic plate impingement occurs when the fracture has united one could offer plate removal. However, in the authors' experience satisfactory plate position is usually possible with careful planning (**Fig. 3**).

Postoperative Care

A volar plaster splint, not including the thumb, is used for 1 week before changing to a distal radius fiberglass cast. The period of immobilization is based on the radiographic assessment of bone union during the follow-up period, which typically lasts between 8 and 10 weeks. The cast is removed after evidence of clinical and radiological signs of fracture healing before commencement of formal hand therapy.

OUTCOMES

Leixnering and colleagues[4] treated 11 patients with scaphoid nonunions of at least 6 months with a volar scaphoid locking plate, 6 of which had previous intramedullary screw fixation and 3 had previous bone grafting. All fractures united at a median interval of 4 months. All patients reported improvements in their symptoms and function. The mean Disabilities of the Arm, Shoulder and Hand score at 6 months postoperatively was 28. Eight patients had regained full function and 4 patients reported minor symptoms such as aching, cold intolerance, or scar tenderness.

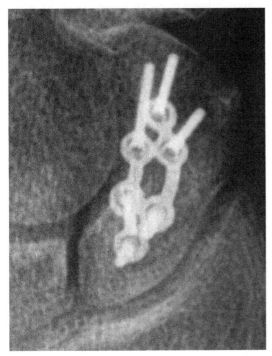

Fig. 3. Intraoperative fluoroscopic image demonstrating optimum plate positioning.

Ghoneim[5] treated 14 scaphoid nonunions without prior surgery using a volar plate. Thirteen patients (93%) achieved union at a mean duration of 3.8 months, with significant improvements in carpal alignment and wrist range of motion. The mean scapholunate angle improved from 61° before surgery to 47° after surgery, and the mean flexion-extension arc of wrist motion improved from 92° to 102°. All except one patient who remained with nonunion reported a good functional rating.

Dodds and colleagues[1] reviewed 20 consecutive scaphoid nonunions with bone loss and humpback deformity treated with this technique. At 6 months postoperatively, 18 patients united (90%) with significant improvements in wrist extension (51° to 62°) and grip strength (32 kg to 39 kg). One nonunion had persistent pain and required further revision. Four patients in this series required plate removal due to impingement against the radius in flexion 1 year after the index procedure.

DISCUSSION

The challenges to scaphoid healing are compounded by the dynamic nature of nonunions, which reduce their healing potential as time passes.[17] Healing declines markedly with increased gapping, fragment separation from the original fracture site, gradual cyst formation, and bone loss.[18] The problems that must be solved include the replacement of necrotic tissue with an osteoconductive matrix and rigid fixation of the healing bones to allow vascular ingrowth and cutting cone penetration. Scaphoid nonunions continue to be challenging and can present notable functional consequences for patients. Many studies of scaphoid nonunion surgery focus on the nature of the bone graft used, such as free versus pedicled vascularized grafts, nonvascularised versus vascularized grafts, and structural versus nonstructural grafts.[19–21] However, few clinical studies place emphasis on the absolute stability of the internal fixation.[14] Although bone grafting is an integral part of nonunion treatment, it is the only one element of the multifactorial reasons that cause nonunions to develop.

Buttress plating offers an additional tool in the surgeon's armamentarium for the more complex scaphoid fractures. Previous failed treatment with a headless intramedullary screw frequently leaves little intact cancellous bone available for revision screw fixation in either the proximal or the distal poles. In this scenario, a volar plate offers an alternative method of internal fixation and can use the intact bone at the periphery of both fragments. The volar ligament splitting approach allows relatively straightforward reduction of any fracture deformity, placement of bone graft, and plate application. Adequate bone grafting can be difficult when using headless screws, because the carefully positioned bone graft is prone to extrusion when compression is applied.[22] A volar plate not only stabilizes the scaphoid and maintains the reduction achieved but also prevents the dislodgement of any prepositioned bone graft by the 2 longitudinal posts in the plate design.

SUMMARY

The authors' preferred treatment for complex acute scaphoid fractures, particularly those with significant comminution and bone loss, and revision cases of complex scaphoid waist nonunions is open reduction and internal fixation using a volar buttress plate. We use volar distal metaphyseal radial cancellous graft through a small cortical window when required, to enable a single-incision approach. This not only offers excellent visualization and assessment of fracture deformity and bone loss, but also facilitates anatomic reduction, bone graft positioning, and placement of a rigid construct in order to resist the powerful flexion and rotational forces at the scaphoid waist. This technique offers an alternative reconstructive option for challenging scaphoid injuries.

REFERENCES

1. Dodds SD, Williams JB, Seiter M, et al. Lessons learned from volar plate fixation of scaphoid fracture nonunions. J Hand Surg Br 2018;43(1):57–65.

2. Kawamura K, Chung KC. Treatment of scaphoid fractures and nonunions. J Hand Surg Am 2008; 33(6):988–97.

3. Henry M. Collapsed scaphoid non-union with dorsal intercalated segment instability and avascular necrosis treated by vascularised wedge-shaped bone graft and fixation. J Hand Surg Br 2007; 32(2):148–54.

4. Leixnering M, Pezzei C, Weninger P, et al. First experiences with a new adjustable plate for osteosynthesis of scaphoid nonunions. J Trauma 2011;71(4):933–8.

5. Ghoneim A. The unstable nonunited scaphoid waist fracture: results of treatment by open reduction, anterior wedge grafting, and internal fixation by volar buttress plate. J Hand Surg Am 2011;36(1):17–24.

6. Buijze GA, Ochtman L, Ring D. Management of scaphoid nonunion. J Hand Surg Am 2012;37(5): 1095–100 [quiz: 1101].

7. Tambe AD, Cutler L, Stilwell J, et al. Scaphoid nonunion: the role of vascularized grafting in recalcitrant non-unions of the scaphoid. J Hand Surg Br 2006; 31(2):185–90.

8. Shah J, Jones WA. Factors affecting the outcome in 50 cases of scaphoid nonunion treated with Herbert screw fixation. J Hand Surg Br 1998;23(5):680–5.

9. Dacho AK, Baumeister S, Germann G, et al. Comparison of proximal row carpectomy and midcarpal arthrodesis for the treatment of scaphoid nonunion advanced collapse (SNAC-wrist) and scapholunate advanced collapse (SLAC-wrist) in stage II. J Plast Reconstr Aesthet Surg 2008;61(10):1210–8.

10. Ender HG. A new method of treating traumatic cysts and pseudoarthrosis of the scaphoid. Unfallheilkunde 1977;80(12):509–13 [in German].

11. Huene DR, Huene DS. Treatment of nonunions of the scaphoid with the Ender compression blade plate system. J Hand Surg Am 1991;16(5):913–22.

12. Braun C, Gross G, Bühren V. Osteosynthesis using a buttress plate–a new principle for stabilizing scaphoid pseudarthroses. Unfallchirurg 1993; 96(1):9–11 [in German].

13. Bain GI, Turow A, Phadnis J. Dorsal plating of unstable scaphoid fractures and nonunions. Tech Hand Up Extrem Surg 2015;19(3):95–100.

14. Dodds SD, Halim A. Scaphoid plate fixation and volar carpal artery vascularized bone graft for recalcitrant scaphoid nonunions. J Hand Surg Am 2016; 41(7):e191–8.

15. Egol KA, Kubiak EN, Fulkerson E, et al. Biomechanics of locked plates and screws. J Orthop Trauma 2004;18(8):488–93.

16. Hagert E, Ferreres A, Garcia-Elias M. Nerve-sparing dorsal and volar approaches to the radiocarpal joint. J Hand Surg Am 2010;35(7):1070–4.

17. Schuind F, Haentjens P, Van Innis F, et al. Prognostic factors in the treatment of carpal scaphoid nonunions. J Hand Surg Am 1999;24(4):761–76.

18. Slade JF, Lozano-Calderon S, Merrell G, et al. Arthroscopic-assisted percutaneous reduction and screw fixation of displaced scaphoid fractures. J Hand Surg Br 2008;33(3):350–4.

19. Straw RG, Davis TRC, Dias JJ. Scaphoid nonunion: treatment with a pedicled vascularized bone graft based on the 1,2 intercompartmental supraretinacular branch of the radial artery. J Hand Surg Br 2002; 27(5):413.

20. Larson AN, Bishop AT, Shin AY. Free medial femoral condyle bone grafting for scaphoid nonunions with humpback deformity and proximal pole avascular necrosis. Tech Hand Up Extrem Surg 2007;11(4): 246–58.

21. Zaidemberg C, Siebert JW, Angrigiani C. A new vascularized bone graft for scaphoid nonunion. J Hand Surg Am 1991;16(3):474–8.

22. Cooney WP, Linscheid RL, Dobyns JH, et al. Scaphoid nonunion: role of anterior interpositional bone grafts. J Hand Surg Am 1988;13(5):635–50.

The Use of the Proximal Hamate as an Autograft for Proximal Pole Scaphoid Fractures
Clinical Outcomes and Biomechanical Implications

Andrea H.W. Chan, MD, FRCSC[a], Bassem T. Elhassan, MD[b],
Nina Suh, MD, FRCSC[c],*

KEYWORDS

- Scaphoid nonunion • Hamate autograft • Scaphoid avascular necrosis
- Proximal pole scaphoid fracture • Fragmented scaphoid fractures

KEY POINTS

- Scaphoid proximal pole fractures remain a surgical challenge because of the high propensity for nonunion, osteonecrosis, and ultimately carpal collapse.
- The proximal pole of the hamate can serve as a replacement arthroplasty in the setting of proximal pole nonunion with collapse, bone loss, and/or osteonecrosis.
- This novel graft provides a local structural autograft solution with minimal donor site morbidity and allows for concurrent scapholunate ligament reconstruction.

INTRODUCTION

Scaphoid proximal pole fractures remain a surgical challenge because of the high propensity for nonunion, osteonecrosis, and ultimately carpal collapse. The proximal 70% to 80% of the scaphoid receives its retrograde blood supply from the dorsal scaphoid branch of the radial artery, which most commonly enters through foramina at the dorsal ridge of the scaphoid waist.[1] Because of this precarious proximal blood supply, it is thought that proximal pole fractures are at high risk of avascular necrosis (AVN) and nonunion. A recent meta-analysis reported that when treated nonoperatively, 34% of acute proximal pole fractures progress to nonunion.[2] This risk is increased to 50% with displacement.[3] In addition, other fracture-specific factors, such as initial displacement, higher energy mechanism of injury, smaller fragment size and fragmentation, and an oblique fracture pattern, have been shown to detrimentally effect the rate of union.[4,5] As a result, various surgical techniques have been developed to address bone loss and optimize vascularity at the fracture site to promote healing; these include vascularized bone grafting (VBG) and nonvascularized bone grafting (NVBG).

Disclosure Statement: No relevant disclosures.
[a] Hand Clinic, Toronto Western Hospital, 399 Bathurst Street, East Wing 2nd Floor, Toronto, Ontario M5T 2S8, Canada; [b] Orthopedic Surgery, Mayo Clinic, 200 1st Street Southwest, Rochester, MN 55905, USA; [c] Roth McFarlane Hand & Upper Limb Centre, University of Western Ontario, St. Joseph's Hospital, 268 Grosvenor Street, Suite D0-215, London, Ontario N6A 4V2, Canada
* Corresponding author.
E-mail address: nina.suh@sjhc.london.on.ca

NVBG,[6] which are typically reserved for proximal pole fractures that maintain their vascularity, have successful union rates ranging from 36% to 89%.[7] Nonvascularized bone donor sites include iliac crest grafts,[8] distal radius autograft,[9] and rib autografts.[10–13] In the setting of previously failed fixation and demonstrable osteonecrosis, VBG have generally demonstrated improved union rates over NVBG options. Reported union rates range from 27% to 100%.[7] Numerous pedicled vascularized and free vascularized graft options exist. Pedicled grafts include the 1,2-intercompartmental suprareticular artery (1,2-ICSRA) dorsal distal radius graft,[14] and the volar carpal artery pedicled pronator quadratus graft.[15] Free vascularized graft options include metatarsal grafts[16] and vascularized osteochondral grafts, such as the medial femoral condyle (MFC) or medial femoral trochlear grafts.[17,18] The femoral vascular grafts have demonstrated consistently high rates of union in the setting of revision surgery for proximal pole nonunions and the presence of osteonecrosis, with studies reporting 84% to 100% union rate.[19–22] They are particularly suitable for situations with carpal collapse and AVN.[19] These techniques, however, pose limitations including donor site morbidity, necessity for microvascular anastomoses, and compromise of the scapholunate (SL) ligament.

Elhassan and colleagues[6] have recently proposed use of the proximal hamate, as a replacement arthroplasty, in the setting of proximal pole nonunions with collapse, bone loss, and/or osteonecrosis. This graft is a nonvascularized osteochondral autograft that maintains its attached volar capitohamate (CH) ligament. It addresses the shortcomings of the previously mentioned graft choices by providing a local solution for osteochondral reconstruction with minimal donor site morbidity, and makes use of the CH ligament for SL ligament reconstruction.

HAMATE ANATOMY

The hamate is a wedge-shaped bone situated on the ulnar aspect of the distal carpal row. The volar hamate serves as the attachment site for the triquetrum-hamate (TH) ligament, a component of the ulnar arm of the arcuate ligament, which functions to counter proximal row flexion and prevent volar intercalated segment instability.[23] Additionally, the distal carpal arch is rigidly constrained in the transverse plane to protect the contents of the carpal tunnel by the transverse carpal ligament that attaches to the volar proximal aspect of the hamate, and the transverse intercarpal ligaments, namely the palmar CH ligament.[23–26] The CH

ligament contributes to the rotational and translational stability of the capitate relative to the hamate and the CH joint is the most stable joint of the wrist comprised of dorsal, deep, and volar components with the deep CH ligament being the stoutest and strongest. Gay and colleagues[27] report that of the wrist ligaments, the dorsal component of the CH ligament shares biomechanical properties most like the dorsal SL ligament. The deep CH ligament is situated at the central axis of rotation and is the primary stabilizer against dorsal translation and rotation, whereas the dorsal ligament is situated distal to the central axis and acts as the primary stabilizer for palmar translation and rotation.[25] The volar component is located at the same central level as the deep component and is stronger than the dorsal contribution,[25] playing a critical role in dorsopalmar stability in the transverse plane.[24] Ritt and colleagues[25] did caution against disruption of the dorsal CH ligament in the setting of a radical carpal boss wedge osteotomy because of the risk of instability. However, the distal row is highly constrained compared with the proximal row[28] and although isolated cadaveric dorsopalmar motion at the CH joint is upward of 17°,[29] this joint motion is constrained to 9° to 10° in in vivo studies demonstrating that there are multiple other stabilizers of the ulnar midcarpus.[30,31]

The hamate is well-vascularized with a consistent dorsal and volar blood supply from the middle transverse carpal arch, and the terminal branches of the anterior interosseous artery and ulnar recurrent artery, respectively.[32] The hook of the hamate also receives blood supply medially from the ulnar recurrent artery.[33,34] AVN of the hamate is rare with only 12 cases reported. The two locations at most risk of developing AVN based on the blood supply are the proximal pole and hook of hamate. Because the proximal pole relies solely on intraosseous supply from the dorsal transverse carpal arch that enters the bone more distally,[33] harvest of the proximal pole would likely not compromise the blood supply to the remaining hamate, thus making this location favorable for a local graft harvest.

A recent anthropometric cadaveric study was undertaken to assess the utility of the proximal hamate as a complete osteochondral graft for this purpose.[35] It was concluded that wrists with an ideal fit had a radial-ulnar proximal hamate fragment and proximal third scaphoid pole width of less than 10 mm, and scaphoid dorsal-volar width less than 16 mm. Thirty-three percent (9/29) of the grafted wrists demonstrated poor fit (>1 mm surface mismatch) in this study. In general, the hamate graft was wider than the scaphoid in the radial-ulnar dimension with 52% of the specimens demonstrating greater width specifically at the dorsal radioscaphoid surface. It is at this dorsal-radial surface of the distal radius in which impaction of the hamate graft occurred in six of the nine poor-fitting specimens. This finding may necessitate intraoperative contouring of the graft at the dorsal radial corner and possibly obtaining preoperative computed tomography (CT) imaging to assess donor and recipient harvest site morphology and fit.

Harley and colleagues[36] studied the biomechanical effect of hamate proximal pole excision in the setting of proximal hamate arthrosis and type II lunates. They concluded that 2.4-mm resection of the proximal hamate was required to completely off-load the hamatolunate articulation. They found the joint forces and articular area across the TH articulation was not significantly altered following this height of proximal hamate excision. In Wu and colleagues'[35] anthropometric study, the average height of proximal hamate resection for use of proximal pole of scaphoid reconstruction was 9.3 mm, far exceeding the amount excised in Harley and colleagues'[36] study. The risk with this resection is disruption of the TH ligament and resultant palmar midcarpal instability. In Elhassan and colleagues'[6] case report, however, this ligament was specifically protected and reinforced with suture anchor repair. No signs of midcarpal instability were identified at the time of the final 3.5-year follow-up. A recent cadaveric biomechanical study[37] published consistent results, demonstrating no significant changes in proximal or midcarpal kinematics following proximal hamate osteotomy at the level of the hook.

SURGICAL TECHNIQUE

The patient is positioned supine with the operative limb on an arm board. An upper arm unsterile tourniquet is placed after obtaining regional anesthesia. A longitudinal skin incision is performed along the dorsum of the wrist and the carpus is accessed via a dorsal ligament-sparing capsulotomy.[38] Maintenance of the integrity of the dorsal intercarpal ligament is important for later SL reconstruction. The proximal pole of the scaphoid and the articular cartilage of the radioscaphoid and radiolunate joints are inspected. The presence of arthritis in these locations is a relative contraindication to replacement arthroplasty using the proximal hamate, and consideration should be made for proceeding with a salvage procedure rather than a joint-preserving procedure. Using an osteotome, the necrotic proximal pole of the scaphoid is then completely resected until punctate bleeding is visualized within the distally remaining scaphoid.

The length, width, and depth of the proximal scaphoid deficit is then measured.

The hamate proximal pole is then visualized at the distal-ulnar extent of the capsulotomy. The previously measured height and width of the proximal scaphoid pole deficit is marked on the proximal hamate pole (**Fig. 1**) and an osteotomy is performed with a small osteotome at the level of the hamate mirroring measurements of the proximal scaphoid pole deficit. This cut surface serves as the interface to the cut scaphoid surface of the remaining distal scaphoid pole. Before osteotomizing the hamate, it is imperative to identify and protect the volar CH ligament because this serves to reconstruct the SL ligament. Additionally, the TH ligament should be identified and protected (**Fig. 2**A). If there is any concern that the TH ligament has been disrupted, it is prudent to repair this to avoid risk of future midcarpal instability. A retractor is placed between the hamate and triquetrum, ensuring the osteotome does not traverse radially through the hamate toward the CH ligament. The hamate fragment is harvested along with the attached volar CH ligament and this fragment is then flipped 180° such that the CH ligament stump is dorsal and the CH articulation forms an articulation with the lunate (**Fig. 2**B). This graft is subsequently placed in the proximal scaphoid deficit (**Fig. 3**A) and temporarily secured within its location with a Kirschner wire. The size of the graft is inspected to ensure appropriate fit between it and the cut surface of the remaining distal scaphoid, at the SL and scaphocapitate articulations, and with the scaphoid facet of the distal radius. The graft's bony edges are trimmed in situ if there is overhang or impingement present, particularly along the dorsal radial aspect of the radioscaphoid articulation. Once the graft is in a

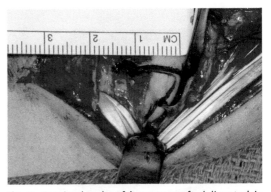

Fig. 1. Proximal pole of hamate graft delineated in purple, before harvesting. The height of hamate harvested should match the height of the cut surface of the remaining distal scaphoid once the proximal pole has been excised. (*Courtesy of* B. Elhassan, MD, Rochester, MN.)

A **B**

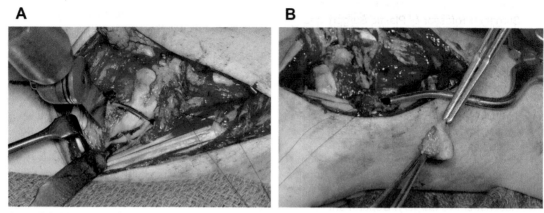

Fig. 2. (*A*) Osteotomy of proximal hamate pole. Retractors are placed to protect the triquetral-hamate ligament. (*B*) The harvested proximal pole of hamate is flipped 180° to demonstrate the attached volar capitohamate ligament, which is held by the lower forceps. (*Courtesy of* B. Elhassan, MD, Rochester, MN.)

satisfactory position and acceptable fit has been obtained, a Kirschner derotation wire is placed across the graft and into the scaphoid. Following this, fluoroscopic-guided fixation is achieved using a buried antegrade single headless compression screw placed down the central axis of the scaphoid. The derotation wire and temporary reduction wire are then removed.

Attention is next turned to the SL reconstruction (**Fig. 3**B). First, the lunate is reduced and held in a neutral position using a retrograde smooth Kirschner wire placed from the capitate into the lunate. This wire configuration, rather than an SL or scaphocapitate wire, is preferentially chosen in this situation to avoid multiple wire placements into the scaphoid and/or hamate graft. This wire is retained to maintain reduction. Following carpal reduction, the CH ligament attached to the hamate graft is then repaired to the stump of the SL ligament on the lunate using a 2–0 nonabsorbable

suture. The SL reconstruction is then reinforced with a distally based strip of the dorsal intercarpal ligament. The capitate-to-lunate Kirschner wire is cut below the level of the skin, and the capsule, extensor retinaculum, subcutaneous tissues, and skin are closed in layers.

POSTOPERATIVE

A below-elbow thumb spica splint is applied for 2 weeks, followed by application of a below-elbow thumb spica cast for at least 6–8 weeks, or until bony union is achieved as determined by postoperative CT scan initially ordered at the 6- to 8-week mark. Bony union is achieved once bridging trabecular bone is observed in more than 50% of the longitudinal sagittal and coronal CT cuts.[39,40] At the time of CT-confirmed union, the capitolunate Kirschner wire is removed, the cast is discontinued, and therapy is initiated.

A **B**

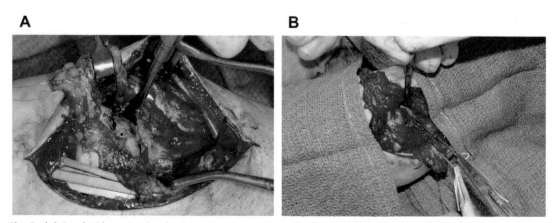

Fig. 3. (*A*) Scaphoid proximal pole reconstruction with proximal pole of hamate placed. The asterisk represents the remaining scaphoid distal pole and the black dot represents the capitohamate ligament, which is used to reconstruct the scapholunate ligament. (*B*) Nonabsorbable sutures are attached to the capitohamate ligament in preparation for scapholunate ligament reconstruction. (*Courtesy of* B. Elhassan, MD, Rochester, MN.)

RESULTS

To date, only one single case study exists regarding the use of the hamate proximal pole for scaphoid proximal pole reconstruction. At 3.5-year postoperative, this patient demonstrated an excellent Mayo Wrist Score, a 120° arc of wrist flexion-extension, full pronosupination, and comparable grip strength to the nonoperative limb. Postoperative radiographs taken at 3-year postoperative demonstrated union and minimal arthritis (**Fig. 4**). He returned to full work duties as a carpenter.[6]

DISCUSSION

Achieving surgical union of the proximal pole is challenging, particularly in the presence of unsalvageable fragmentation, carpal collapse, or AVN. Several surgical techniques have been described including VBG and NVBG options. Literature suggests that VBGs confer higher proximal pole union rates than NVGBs in these challenging settings. A meta-analysis by Merrell and colleagues[41] reported a union rate of 47% following use of NVBG in the setting of nonunion and proximal pole AVN, versus 88% with use of VBG. Goldberg

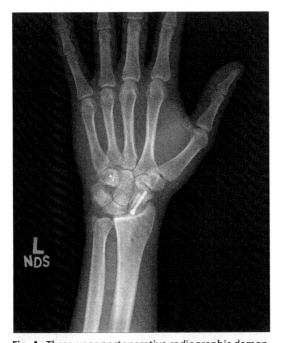

Fig. 4. Three-year postoperative radiographic demonstration of successful scaphoid union. Note the antegrade compression screw used for the scaphoid reconstruction, and the hamate-based suture anchor used for triquetrum-hamate ligament reinforcement after graft harvest. (*Courtesy of* B. Elhassan, MD, Rochester, MN.)

and colleagues[42] hypothesize VBG success is related to higher rates of osteocyte survival that minimizes creeping substitution and graft resorption. Despite these results, however, the outcomes following VBGs are variable and graft selection seems to be related to the graft type, proximal pole size, and the presence of scaphoid collapse or AVN.

Both pedicled and free vascularized grafts have been described. By far, the most commonly used pedicled graft is the 1,2-ICSRA.[14] This graft demonstrates rates of union ranging from 12% to 100% in the setting of proximal pole fractures with AVN raising concern that this graft success is not universal.[43] In fact, Chang and colleagues[44] suggested that the 1,2-ICSRA graft should be contraindicated in the setting of small or collapsed proximal pole fractures. The presence of carpal collapse and/or humpback deformity increases the risk of nonunion suggesting that restoration of scaphoid geometry with a use of a structural graft is required for successful union.[22,45,46] Pedicled inlay VBGs, such as the 1,2-ICSRA, are limited by their size and ability to correct deformity or dorsal intercalated segmental instability.[45] Henry[47] reported a 71% union rate using the 1,2-ICSRA inlay volar graft and found that failures were associated with preoperative humpback deformities. Chang and colleagues[44] found the presence of proximal pole AVN decreased the union rate from 91% to 50% and increased time to union from 14 weeks to 18 weeks, despite using an inlay 1,2-ICSRA graft. In this study, the odds ratio of nonunion in the setting of AVN was significantly high at 9.6. Straw and colleagues[48] also attributed their low rate of union (27%) following 1,2-ICSRA grafting to the inclusion of a high number of patients with proximal pole AVN (16/22). The use of the pedicled 1,2-ICSRA therefore does not provide optimal or consistent results in the setting of small proximal pole fractures with AVN or proximal pole fractures associated with carpal collapse.

The MFC VBG is a free structural vascularized graft that has received recent attention. A meta-analysis demonstrated that the MFC VBG had the best healing potential in the setting of proximal pole AVN at 97.4% compared with all other vascularized flaps analyzed, whereas the worst healing potential was seen in association with the 1,2-ICSRA VBG at 79.2%.[49] The MFC provides a large osteochondral alternative to the 1,2-ICSRA that is ideal in the setting of proximal pole AVN and carpal collapse.[45,49] When compared with the 1,2-ICSRA, the MFC graft demonstrated earlier time to union (median, 13 weeks vs 19 weeks) and better ability to restore the interscaphoid and SL angles (average, 57° to 32° and 70° to 57°, respectively).[22]

The MFC graft, however, has an inherent risk of donor site morbidity. Mehio and colleagues[50] reported an overall complication rate of 18.6%, with the most common complication being paraesthesias or numbness in the saphenous nerve distribution at 8%. Other complications included infection (4%), hematoma (2.7%), and pain. Jones and colleagues[22] reported knee discomfort for an average 6-week postoperative, and Mehio and colleagues[50] reported that 4% of patients experienced donor site pain lasting more than 3 months. In addition to donor site morbidity, a microvascular skill set is required to perform an end-to-side anastomosis to the radial artery and end-to-end anastomosis to the venae comitantes. Lastly, this graft does not address reconstruction of the SL ligament.

Traditional NVBG options include corticocancellous graft from the iliac crest[8] and distal radius.[9] In the setting of a deficient proximal pole caused by AVN or fragmentation, nonvascularized structural osteochondral grafts, such as that from the rib[10] and hamate,[6] have been used as replacement arthroplasties. Traditional NVBGs have demonstrated lower union rates in the setting of proximal pole fractures and AVN, which are lower than VBGs.[41] In general, structural NVBG has been reserved for proximal pole nonunions wherein the vascular supply has not been compromised.[7] However, it has been recently demonstrated that union rates may be independent of proximal scaphoid pole viability.[51] Although more than 50% of patients in this study had histologic evidence of trabecular necrosis at the scaphoid nonunion site, there was no association to intraoperative punctate bleeding, preoperative MRI signal, or fracture location. In fact, 91% of these patients also demonstrated active remodeling and 88% viable connective tissue indicating that complete necrosis was absent in this cohort of patients. Of these patients, 97% went on to successful union with nonvascularized iliac crest or distal radius autograft, suggesting that not only is the preoperative prediction of viability unreliable, but that NVBG is still a reasonable option even when vascularity is questioned.

Rib costochondral autograft has been used for the reconstruction of the unsalvageable proximal scaphoid pole and has demonstrated promising results. Four case series are reported in the literature.[11–13,52] Nearly all patients are reported to have functional improvement, and no scaphoids failed to heal or proceed on to carpal collapse within the 15 months to 64 months of recorded follow-up. Disadvantages of this technique, however, include donor site morbidity including chest wall surgical site scar and theoretic risk of pneumothorax or pleural tears.

The proximal hamate osteochondral nonvascularized graft offers a promising alternative to the commonly used VBGs and NVBGs for scaphoid proximal pole nonunions. First, it addresses the donor morbidity site issues by using the same operative approach without compromising carpal stability. Second, it provides a structural osteochondral option, of morphologic similarity to the proximal pole, to act as a replacement arthroplasty when there is unreconstructable proximal pole fragmentation, collapse, and necrosis. Third, the technique reconstructs the SL ligament using the attached CH ligament, which is particularly important in cases wherein dorsal intercalated segmental instability correction is necessitated. Furthermore, the CH ligament closely resembles the SL ligament in its biomechanical properties. Lastly, the proximal hamate graft provides a more universal option, because a specialized microvascular skill set is not required.

Currently, only a single case study[6] exists regarding the use of ipsilateral hamate proximal pole autograft for proximal scaphoid pole reconstruction. Further larger-scale studies are needed to demonstrate consistent favorable short- and long-term functional outcomes and radiographic healing following the use of the proximal hamate graft for scaphoid proximal pole nonunions. Additionally, minimal literature exists regarding specific anatomic locations of the hamate intercarpal ligaments. Such studies would be beneficial to determine size limitations of this graft option.

SUMMARY

The use of the nonvascularized hamate proximal pole for proximal pole scaphoid fractures is a promising alternative to existing options, particularly when the proximal pole is irreparable, such as in the case of AVN or pole comminution. The main advantages of this technique are that it offers a local well-fitted osteochondral graft option with minimal known donor site morbidity and mitigates the need for microvascular anastomoses. Additionally, it provides a robust ligament to reconstruct the SL articulation and offers structural capability to restore carpal collapse. Further longer-term functional outcome and radiographic studies are required to confirm the clinical success of this procedure, and biomechanical studies will help to elucidate the impact of this graft harvest on midcarpal kinematics and stability.

REFERENCES

1. Gelberman RH, Menon J. The vascularity of the scaphoid bone. J Hand Surg Am 1980;5(5):508–13.

2. Eastley N, Singh H, Dias JJ, et al. Union rates after proximal scaphoid fractures; meta-analyses and review of available evidence. J Hand Surg Eur Vol 2013;38(8):888–97.

3. Düppe H, Johnell O, Lundborg G, et al. Long-term results of fracture of the scaphoid. A follow-up study of more than thirty years. J Bone Joint Surg Am 1994;76(2):249–52.

4. Brogan DM, Moran SL, Shin AY. Outcomes of open reduction and internal fixation of acute proximal pole scaphoid fractures. Hand (N Y) 2015;10(2): 227–32.

5. Luchetti TJ, Hedroug Y, Fernandez JJ, et al. The morphology of proximal pole scaphoid fractures: implications for optimal screw placement. J Hand Surg Eur Vol 2018;43(1):73–9.

6. Elhassan B, Noureldin M, Kakar S. Proximal scaphoid pole reconstruction utilizing ipsilateral proximal hamate autograft. Hand (N Y) 2016;11(4): 495–9.

7. Steinmann SP, Adams JE. Scaphoid fractures and nonunions: diagnosis and treatment. J Orthop Sci 2006;11(4):424–31.

8. Robbins RR, Ridge O, Carter PR. Iliac crest bone grafting and Herbert screw fixation of nonunions of the scaphoid with avascular proximal poles. J Hand Surg Am 1995;20(5):818–31.

9. Shah J, Jones WA. Factors affecting the outcome in 50 cases of scaphoid nonunion treated with Herbert screw fixation. J Hand Surg Br 1998;23(5):680–5.

10. Sandow MJ. Costo-osteochondral grafts in the wrist. Tech Hand Up Extrem Surg 2001;5(3):165–72.

11. Veitch S, Blake SM, David H. Proximal scaphoid rib graft arthroplasty. J Bone Joint Surg Br 2007;89(2): 196–201.

12. Lanzetta M. Scaphoid reconstruction by a free vascularized osteochondral graft from the rib: a case report. Microsurgery 2009;29(5):420–4.

13. Yao J, Read B, Hentz VR. The fragmented proximal pole scaphoid nonunion treated with rib autograft: case series and review of the literature. J Hand Surg Am 2013;38(11):2188–92.

14. Zaidemberg C, Siebert JW, Angrigiani C. A new vascularized bone graft for scaphoid nonunion. J Hand Surg Am 1991;16(3):474–8.

15. Kuhlmann JN, Mimoun M, Boabighi A, et al. Vascularized bone graft pedicled on the volar carpal artery for non-union of the scaphoid. J Hand Surg Br 1987; 12(2):203–10.

16. del Pinal F, Klausmeyer M, Moraleda E, et al. Vascularized graft from the metatarsal base for reconstructing major osteochondral distal radius defects. J Hand Surg Am 2013;38(10):1883–95.

17. Kazmers NH, Thibaudeau S, Levin LS. A scapholunate ligament-sparing technique utilizing the medial femoral condyle corticocancellous free flap to reconstruct scaphoid nonunions with proximal pole avascular necrosis. J Hand Surg Am 2016;41(9):e309–15.

18. Burger HK, Windhofer C, Gaggl AJ, et al. Vascularized medial femoral trochlea osteocartilaginous flap reconstruction of proximal pole scaphoid nonunions. J Hand Surg Am 2013;38(4):690–700.

19. Pulos N, Kollitz KM, Bishop AT, et al. Free vascularized medial femoral condyle bone graft after failed scaphoid nonunion surgery. J Bone Joint Surg Am 2018;100(16):1379–86.

20. Aibinder WR, Wagner ER, Bishop AT, et al. Bone grafting for scaphoid nonunions: is free vascularized bone grafting superior for scaphoid nonunion? Hand (N Y) 2019;14(2):217–22.

21. Doi K, Oda T, Soo-Heong T, et al. Free vascularized bone graft for nonunion of the scaphoid. J Hand Surg Am 2000;25(3):507–19.

22. Jones DB, Bürger H, Bishop AT, et al. Treatment of scaphoid waist nonunions with an avascular proximal pole and carpal collapse. A comparison of two vascularized bone grafts. J Bone Joint Surg Am 2008;90(12):2616–25.

23. Garcia-Elias M, Lluch AL. Wrist instabilities, misalignments, and dislocations. In: Wolfe SW, Hotchkiss RN, Pederson WC, et al, editors. Green's operative hand surgery, vol. 1, 7th edition. Philadelphia: Elsevier; 2017. p. 418–78.

24. Garcia-Elias M, An KN, Cooney WP, et al. Stability of the transverse carpal arch: an experimental study. J Hand Surg Am 1989;14(2 Pt 1):277–82.

25. Ritt MJ, Berger RA, Kauer JM. The gross and histologic anatomy of the ligaments of the capitohamate joint. J Hand Surg Am 1996;21(6):1022–8.

26. Berger RA. The ligaments of the wrist. A current overview of anatomy with considerations of their potential functions. Hand Clin 1997;13(1):63–82.

27. Gay AM, Thoreson A, Berger RA. Biomechanical comparison of the hand-based transplant used in bone-tissue-bone scapho-lunate ligament reconstruction. Chir Main 2014;33(1):23–8.

28. Berger RA, Garcia-Elias M. General anatomy of the wrist. In: An KN, Berger RA, Cooney WP, editors. Biomechanics of the wrist joint. New York: Springer Verlag; 1991. p. 1–22.

29. Kaplan EB, Taleisnik J. The wrist. In: Spinner M, editor. Kaplan's functional and surgical anatomy of the hand. 3rd edition. Philadelphia: J.B. Lippincott Company; 1984. p. 153–201.

30. de Lange A, Kauer JM, Huiskes R. Kinematic behavior of the human wrist joint: a roentgen-stereophotogrammetric analysis. J Orthop Res 1985;3(1):56–64.

31. Ruby LK, Cooney WP 3rd, An KN, et al. Relative motion of selected carpal bones: a kinematic analysis of the normal wrist. J Hand Surg Am 1988;13(1):1–10.

32. Rozen WM, Niumsawatt V, Ross R, et al. The vascular basis of the hemi-hamate osteochondral

free flap. Part 1: vascular anatomy and clinical correlation. Surg Radiol Anat 2013;35(7):585–94.

33. Peters SJ, Verstappen C, Degreef I, et al. Avascular necrosis of the hamate: three cases and review of the literature. J Wrist Surg 2014;3(4):269–74.

34. Freedman DM, Botte MJ, Gelberman RH. Vascularity of the carpus. Clin Orthop Relat Res 2001; 383:47–59.

35. Wu K, Padmore C, Lalone E, et al. An anthropometric assessment of the proximal hamate autograft for scaphoid proximal pole reconstruction. J Hand Surg Am 2019;44(1):60.e1-8.

36. Harley BJ, Werner FW, Boles SD, et al. Arthroscopic resection of arthrosis of the proximal hamate: a clinical and biomechanical study. J Hand Surg Am 2004;29(4):661–7.

37. Kakar S, Greene RM, Hewett T, et al. The effect of proximal hamate osteotomy on carpal kinematics for reconstruction of proximal pole scaphoid nonunion with avascular necrosis. Hand (N Y) 2018. https://doi.org/10.1177/1558944718793175.

38. Berger RA, Bishop AT, Bettinger PC. New dorsal capsulotomy for the surgical exposure of the wrist. Ann Plast Surg 1995;35(1):54–9.

39. Suh N, Grewal R. Controversies and best practices for acute scaphoid fracture management. J Hand Surg Eur Vol 2018;43(1):4–12.

40. Singh HP, Forward D, Davis TR, et al. Partial union of acute scaphoid fractures. J Hand Surg Br 2005; 30(5):440–5.

41. Merrell GA, Wolfe SW, Slade JF 3rd. Treatment of scaphoid nonunions: quantitative meta-analysis of the literature. J Hand Surg Am 2002;27(4):685–91.

42. Goldberg VM, Shaffer JW, Field G, et al. Biology of vascularized bone grafts. Orthop Clin North Am 1987;18(2):197–205.

43. Lim TK, Kim HK, Koh KH, et al. Treatment of avascular proximal pole scaphoid nonunions with vascularized distal radius bone grafting. J Hand Surg Am 2013;38(10):1906–12.e1.

44. Chang MA, Bishop AT, Moran SL, et al. The outcomes and complications of 1,2-intercompartmental supraretinacular artery pedicled vascularized bone grafting of scaphoid nonunions. J Hand Surg Am 2006;31(3):387–96.

45. Kakar S, Bishop AT, Shin AY. Role of vascularized bone grafts in the treatment of scaphoid nonunions associated with proximal pole avascular necrosis and carpal collapse. J Hand Surg Am 2011;36(4): 722–5.

46. Jones DB, Rhee PC, Shin AY. Vascularized bone grafts for scaphoid nonunions. J Hand Surg Am 2012;37(5):1090–4.

47. Henry M. Collapsed scaphoid non-union with dorsal intercalated segment instability and avascular necrosis treated by vascularised wedge-shaped bone graft and fixation. J Hand Surg Eur Vol 2007; 32(2):148–54.

48. Straw RG, Davis TR, Dias JJ. Scaphoid nonunion: treatment with a pedicled vascularized bone graft based on the 1,2 intercompartmental supraretinacular branch of the radial artery. J Hand Surg Br 2002;27(5):413.

49. Ditsios K, Konstantinidis I, Agas K, et al. Comparative meta-analysis on the various vascularized bone flaps used for the treatment of scaphoid nonunion. J Orthop Res 2017;35(5):1076–85.

50. Mehio G, Morsy M, Cayci C, et al. Donor site morbidity and functional status following medial femoral condyle flap harvest. Plast Reconstr Surg 2018;142(5):734e–41e.

51. Rancy SK, Swanstrom MM, DiCarlo EF, et al. Success of scaphoid nonunion surgery is independent of proximal pole vascularity. J Hand Surg Eur Vol 2018;43(1):32–40.

52. Sandow MJ. Proximal scaphoid costo-osteochondral replacement arthroplasty. J Hand Surg Br 1998;23(2):201–8.

Arthroscopic Management of Scaphoid Nonunion

Wing-Yee Clara Wong, MBChB, MRCS, FRCSEd (Orth), FHKAM (Orthopaedic Surgery), FHKCOS[a,b,c],
Pak-Cheong Ho, MBBS, FRCS (Edinburg), FHKAM (Orthopaedic Surgery), FHKCOS[a,d,e],*

KEYWORDS

- Arthroscopic bone graft • Scaphoid • Nonunion • Wrist arthroscopy

KEY POINTS

- Surgical treatment of scaphoid nonunion is done to prevent the progression of carpal collapse and arthritis.
- Open techniques using nonvascularized or vascularized bone grafts have their limitations and drawbacks related to compromising local vascularity.
- Minimally invasive techniques have advantages in cases of scaphoid nonunion. The authors think arthroscopic bone grafting represents a major advancement for arthroscopic wrist surgery.
- With proper surgical techniques and experience, high union rates and good clinical outcomes can be achieved.

 Video content accompanies this article at http://www.hand.theclinics.com.

INTRODUCTION

Principles of Surgical Treatments of Scaphoid Nonunion

The natural history of scaphoid nonunion has been well reported.[1-6] Scaphoid nonunion can result in pain, altered wrist kinematics, and motion deficits.[6] Wrist osteoarthritis is likely to develop in untreated nonunions.[1-5] Because most scaphoid fractures occur in young and active individuals, scaphoid nonunion and the development of scaphoid nonunion advanced collapse (SNAC) has the potential to create great functional impairment. The goal is timely restoration of the scaphoid architecture to prevent progression of carpal collapse and arthritis. Despite various surgical techniques, the principles for successful management of scaphoid nonunion are the same: excision of pseudoarthrosis, to interpose fibrous scar and necrotic bone, correction of humpback deformity, bone grafting, and rigid internal stabilization of the proximal and distal scaphoid fragments.

Bone Grafting Options for Nonunions

Nonvascularized bone graft

Bone grafting is the mainstay of operative treatment of scaphoid nonunion. It provides a healing environment with both osteoconductive and osteoinductive ability. It can be nonvascularized or vascularized, especially for nonunions that are more likely to fail such as proximal pole or avascular necrosis. Nonvascularized bone grafting

Disclosure Statement: The authors have no relationship with any commercial company that has a direct financial interest in subject matter or materials discussed in article or with a company making a competing product.
a Faculty of Medicine, The Chinese University of Hong Kong, HKSAR; b Hand Wrist Elbow and Microsurgery Clinic, The Chinese University of Hong Kong Medical Clinic, HKSAR; c The Club Lusitano, 16/F, 16 Ice House Street, Central, Hong Kong SAR; d Prince of Wales Hospital, Alice Ho Miu Ling Nethersole Hospital, Tai Po Hospital; e Division of Hand and Microsurgery, Department of Orthopaedics and Traumatology, Prince of Wales Hospital
* Corresponding author. Prince of Wales Hospital, Room 74034, 5/F, Clinical Science Building, Shatin, HKSAR.
E-mail address: pcho@ort.cuhk.edu.hk

Hand Clin 35 (2019) 295–313
https://doi.org/10.1016/j.hcl.2019.03.003

techniques include inlay grafting, pioneered by Matti[7,8] in 1936 and then modified by Russe[9] in 1960, and intercalated wedge bone graft, by Fisk[10] in 1980 and Fernandez[11] in 1984. Less invasive bone graft techniques, such as trephine bone grafting, were advocated by Maruthainar[12] in 2000 and Leung and colleagues[13] in 2001. Although the union incidence in nonvascularized bone graft as reviewed by Pinder and colleagues[14] was 88%, their series was used more often for nonunions that were more unlikely to fail and so the result of union incidence may be skewed. A meta-analysis performed by Merrell and colleagues[15] revealed that nonvascularized bone grafts could only achieve a 47% union rate in avascular necrosis of the proximal fragment and some reports have noted an incidence as low as 38%.[16]

Vascularized bone graft

The vascularized bone grafting technique provides viable bone and creates an osteogenic potential to promote union. It has an estimated overall union incidence of 92%, as shown in the systemic review by Pinder and colleagues[14] in 2015, and 84.7%, shown in the critical appraisal by Alluri and colleagues.[17] It includes pedicled vascularized bone graft and free vascularized graft. Pedicled vascularized bone grafting can be transferred on a pedicle from the scaphoid tubercle, described by Judet and colleagues[18] in 1972; from the pronator quadratus pedicle, first described by Braun[19] in 1983; from pisiform, described by Kuhlmann and colleagues[20] in 1986; from volar distal radius based on the palmar carpal artery, first described by Kuhlmann and colleagues[21] in 1987; from ulna based on the ulnar artery, described by Guimberteau and Panconi[22] in 1990; from dorsal distal radius based on the 1,2-intercompartmental supraretinacular artery, described by Zaidemberg and colleagues[23] in 1991; from second metacarpal based on the second dorsal metacarpal artery, as suggested by Brunelli in 1991[24] and used by Mathoulin and Brunelli[25] in 1998; and from thumb metacarpal based on the pedicel on the first dorsal metacarpal artery, described by Yuceturk and colleagues[26] in 1997. Free vascularized bone grafting can be from iliac crest, described by Pechlaner and colleagues[27] in 1987; from medial femoral condyle, described by Doi and colleagues[28] in 2000; and from rib described by Veitch and colleagues[29,30] in 2007. Not all reports on the use of vascularized bone graft have been favorable; overall, there is a 16% complication rate. Deep infection, superficial infection, graft extrusion, hardware failure, wrist stiffness, complex regional pain syndrome, and neuropathic pain have been reported.[17,30–34] Although a microsurgical anastomosis is not required with a pedicled vascularized bone graft, reported disadvantages include difficulty in identifying the pedicles after exsanguination,[35] difficulty in adequate visualization of the fracture site reduction, loss of reduction, limited pedicle rotation arc,[35–37] difficulty in obtaining and positioning the graft,[25] limited pedicle length,[22,23] and extensive dissection.[22,35,38] A recent meta-analysis by Ditsios and colleagues[39] showed that free vascularized medial femoral condyle bone grafting was the most successful in its potential to bring vascularity and union of the scaphoid. However, the operation is complex, demands long operation time and microvascular technique, has limitations in postoperative range of motion, and has the complication of ectopic bone formation limiting wrist motion.[40,41] Any type of open surgery has the drawbacks of pain, stiffness, and hypertrophic scar.[34]

Open Procedures and Minimally Invasive Surgeries in Scaphoid Nonunion

Open approaches to the scaphoid have the risk of jeopardizing the residual vascularity, which affects the bone graft union and can damage the capsular and ligamentous structures surrounding the scaphoid, which leads to wrist stiffness. An alternative to open reduction was proposed in 2006 when Slade and Dodds[42] described the techniques that allowed for fracture site debridement; the bone graft was inserted percutaneously and the fracture was fixed rigidly. This minimally invasive approach avoided the common complications of open repair, including hypertrophic scar formation, avascular necrosis, carpal instability, donor site pain, bone graft infection, screw protrusion, and reflex sympathetic dystrophy.[43] It reduced additional soft tissue injury and permitted early restoration of hand function.[42,43] However, the amount of bone graft inserted was limited and repeat bone grafting was required in 12.2% of patients (10 out of 82 scaphoid nonunions).[43]

The Birth of Arthroscopic Bone Grafting

In April 1997, arthroscopic bone grafting (ABG) was first done in a 50-year-old man with scaphoid nonunion after percutaneous screw fixation that had been performed 5 months prior (**Fig. 1**). The fracture was united 3 months after ABG. The patient enjoyed good range of motion, pinch, and grip power. In May 1998, current author P.C. Ho first reported in the 7th Congress of International Federation of Societies for Surgery of the Hand, Vancouver, Canada, on the technique of ABG in osseous defects in 11 cases, including scaphoid nonunion, acute comminuted scaphoid fracture, carpal bone cysts, and triscaphe fusion. Union

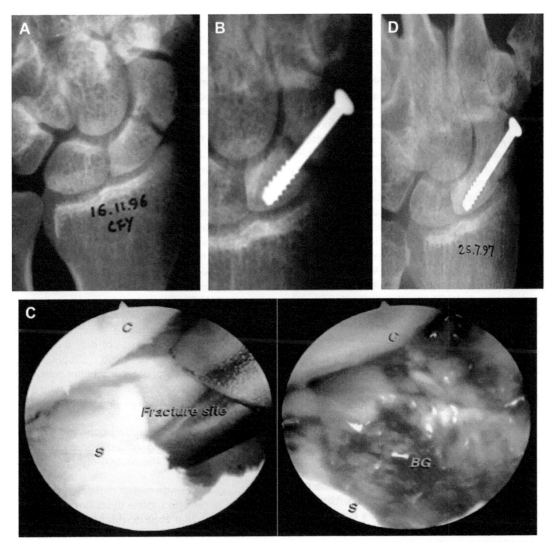

Fig. 1. (*A*) Left scaphoid acute fracture in a 50-year-old man in November 1996. (*B*) 5 months after percutaneous screw fixation. Wide fracture gap was seen. (*C*) ABG was done in Apr 1997. Left is showing impacting the bone graft in the fracture gap; on the right is showing the bone graft in the fracture gap. (*D*) Radiograph showed scaphoid fracture well united at 3 months. BG, bone graft.

was achieved in all patients at an average of 3.4 months. Since then, ABG is the authors' primary standard treatment in all uncomplicated scaphoid delayed and nonunion cases, including those with features of avascular necrosis.

RATIONALE OF ARTHROSCOPIC BONE GRAFTING
Why Is Scaphoid Fracture Susceptible to Nonunion and How Does Arthroscopic Bone Grafting Help Nonunion to Heal?

Main deforming forces across the scaphoid fracture: shearing, bending, and pronation forces
Scaphoid fracture can be inherently unstable. It acts as a long level arm and is the only carpal bone linking the proximal and distal carpal rows. Smith and colleagues[44] demonstrated in 5 cadaveric specimens that there was increased motion of the distal scaphoid fragment but decreased motion of the proximal fragment during wrist motion. This creates significant multiplanar interfragmentary motion and shearing forces across the 2 scaphoid fragments. Because of the complex osseous-capsular-ligamentous construct of scaphoid, bending and pronation forces affect the distal scaphoid fragment, resulting in flexion and pronation deformity, and collapse of the scaphoid.[44,45] Both the interfragmentary motions, scaphoid collapse and flexion or pronation deformity, affect the kinematics of the other carpal bones, which further exaggerates the fracture instability.[44]

Absolute stability is essential for scaphoid fracture healing

Approximately 75% of the surface of the scaphoid is covered with cartilage, forming articulation with adjacent bones.[46,47] There are only tiny patches of periosteum on the nonarticular and nonligamentous attached surfaces.[48] With limited periosteum and the lack of the periosteal source of chondrogenic and osteoblastic cells, scaphoid fractures do not easily make callus. Synovial fluid may also dilute the fracture hematoma and inflammatory and osteogenic cells.[49] Synovial fluid contains inhibitors of osteoblast proliferation, which may retard callus formation.[50–52] Scaphoid fractures mainly rely on primary bone healing via cutting cones bridging the fracture and Haversian remodeling. Direct bone contact and absolute fracture stability are, therefore, crucial. With the consequence of its poor ability to form callus to provide initial structural stability, rigid stability should also be maintained for a sufficient period during the fracture healing process.

Tenuous vascularity of the scaphoid

Vascular supply to the scaphoid plays a critical role in fracture healing. Branches of the radial artery entering through the distal dorsal ridge supply 70% to 80% of the intraosseous vascularity and whole proximal pole.[53] The large volume of bone that depends on a single intraosseous vessel poses a high risk of avascular necrosis and fracture nonunion.[54]

With the inherent instability and precarious vascularity at the scaphoid fracture site, if the fracture stability is not secured, primary bone healing is difficult. Without periosteum around the fracture site, secondary bone healing can still occur and callus can still be formed from the chondrogenic and osteoblastic cells coming from the endosteum, trabeculae, and Haversian systems proximal and distal to the fracture.[48] However, this is not as favorable as primary bone healing. The continuous motion would cause vascular perforators to recede from the fracture site and the avascular zone would be widened. With increased cell death, the bone matrix would be absorbed and replaced by avascular bone cysts.[42] The secondary bone healing would then decline markedly, with increased gapping and necrotic tissue interposed. Hence, nonunion would definitely occur.

How Does Arthroscopic Bone Grafting Promote Scaphoid Union?

- After adequate arthroscopic debridement, and removal of the interposed fibrous tissue and sclerotic avascular bone, flexion and pronation deformity can be corrected by closed means.
- After initial pinning across the fracture gap, iliac crest cancellous bone graft is impacted to fill up the gap. The fracture gap is larger than expected after the scaphoid collapse and deformity are corrected. Restoring the normal scaphoid length and alignment helps restore the normal tautness of the surrounding ligaments and the kinematics of the whole wrist, which may lessen the mobility of the fracture.
- The volume of the bone graft to be inserted is also more than expected. It should be at least 3 to 5 times that of the defect as the cancellous bone graft is impacted and compressed tightly to the fracture defect. The firm and impacted bone graft helps maintain the scaphoid length and provide immediate structure stability.
- Despite the lack of periosteum for secondary bone healing, the dense autologous cancellous bone graft serves not only a osteoconduction role but also supplies high concentrations of osteoprogenitor cells, osteoblasts, osteocytes, and chemotactic mitogens to promote graft integration and bone growth.
- The dense and impacted bone graft scaffold and the overlying added fibrous glue may help to prevent the dilution effect of synovial fluid.
- In nonunion with higher mobility, the fracture site is resorbed, bone cysts are formed, and the avascular zone is widened. Failure of mechanical loading can result in further decrease in bone density and biomaterial stiffness of the whole scaphoid as time passes.[5,44,55] Screw purchase in the soft and small bone fragments would be insufficient to provide sufficient fracture stability. However, impacted cancellous bone graft helps give additional structural support. The healing biology of cancellous bone graft occurs through the dual processes of resorption and substitution. Absolute stability for cutting cones to pass through the fracture site is not necessary. Therefore, screw compression characteristics are not essential. Multiple Kirschner (K)-wires across the fracture site can also be sufficient to resist the bending, pronation, and shearing forces during the process of fracture healing.
- Scaphoid is an almost entire intraarticular bone. It is logical and reasonable to work on the scaphoid arthroscopically. In the midcarpal joint (MCJt), the gentle curvature of the scaphoid body enables a stable and spacious

platform for the necessary arthroscopic bone work on it.

- Arthroscopic surgery helps preserve the tenuous vascularity around the scaphoid.

Contraindications

Limitations do exist for ABG, including

1. Long-standing scaphoid nonunion with significant carpal collapse cannot be adequately corrected after arthroscopic fibrosis release and close reduction.
2. Severe SNAC wrist changes likely preclude good outcome from scaphoid union after bone grafting.

Avascular necrosis is not an absolute contraindication, though the chance of persistent nonunion is higher than in cases with good intraoperation bone bleeding. Arthrofibrosis that causes difficult access by the arthroscope may be a relative contraindication. Nevertheless, with experience, patience, and the use of a smaller arthroscope, most fibrotic joints can be loosened up gradually by careful arthroscopic debridement and dilation to provide adequate working space for subsequent bone works.

SURGICAL TECHNIQUES
Setup

The patient is put in supine position. The operated arm is supported on a hand table. Either side of the iliac crest is draped for bone graft harvesting. An arm tourniquet is applied and inflated only if necessary. Vertical traction of 4 to 6 kg force is applied through plastic finger traps to the index, middle, and ring fingers. A bag of 3 L of normal saline solution is hung up at about 1.5 m height for continuous joint instillation. An infusion pump is not necessary and potentially causes fluid extravasation.

Arthroscopic Surveillance

The arthroscopic surveillance step can be performed under portal site local anesthesia.[56] The patient is awake and watching the arthroscopy monitor (**Fig. 2**). This is helpful for the patients in understanding their disease condition, severity, prognosis, and the treatment choices, so that they comply with subsequent rehabilitation. Adrenaline 1:200,000 dilution is injected only to the portal site skin to reduce operative bleeding (**Fig. 3**). The authors routinely inspect both the radiocarpal joint (RCJt) and the MCJt through the 3-4 portal and midcarpal radial (MCR) portals, respectively, with a 1.9-mm arthroscope (**Fig. 4**).

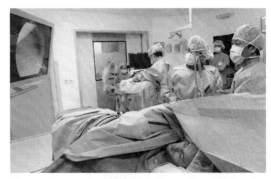

Fig. 2. The patient was awake and watching the arthroscopy monitor during the wrist arthroscopy.

Any accompanying chondral lesion related to SNAC wrist changes should be documented because it affects the prognosis and choice of procedure. The dorsal rim of radial styloid is a common site of occurrence of early SNAC wrist changes and is best observed through the 4-5 portal. Any associated synovitis at this area may obscure the observation of true cartilage condition and must be removed. Unless it is a very proximal

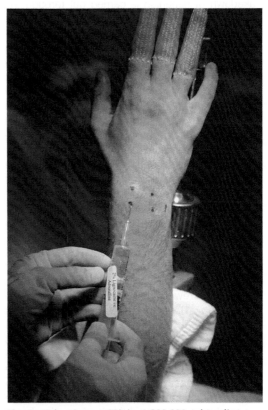

Fig. 3. Xylocaine at 2% in 1:200,000 adrenaline was injected only to the portal site skin to reduce operative bleeding.

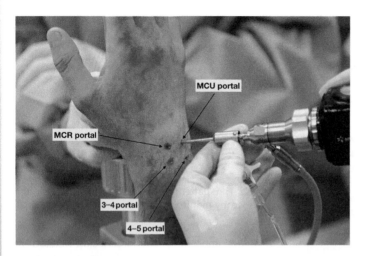

Fig. 4. The 3-4 portal is used for inspecting the RCJt and doing the radial styloidectomy, the 4-5 portal is used for clear inspection of the cartilage status of dorsal aspect of scaphoid fossa and radial styloid, the MCR portal is used for bone graft insertion, and the midcarpal ulnar (MCU) portal may also be used as a viewing portal.

fracture, it is usually not seen from the RCJt. The fracture is obscured by the capsular reflection, which helps contain subsequent bone grafting implanted through the MCJt.

Takedown of Nonunion

Takedown of nonunion is carried out through the MCJt. The MCR is the working portal, whereas the midcarpal ulnar (MCU) is for viewing. The MCR portal is more difficult to develop and the working space through the MCR portal is narrower as a result of fracture malalignment, bone spurs at the nonunion site, intraarticular fibrosis, and secondary capsular contracture. It is, however, the best portal for takedown of the fibrosis. In the distal-third nonunion, scaphoid-trapezium-trapezoid (STT) portal is frequently required to provide a more direct access (**Fig. 5**). The nonunion is located by a cleavage line in the scaphoid articular surface or by a frank gapping (**Fig. 6**).

The fracture gap is directly palpated with a probe inserted through the MCR portal. Healing bone is usually found in the center of the fracture. If stable bony tissue is encountered after initial debridement of the overlying fibrous tissue or there is lack of mobility at the fracture site by probing, simple screw fixation or even casting may suffice (Video 1). If a frank bony defect is encountered, it is curetted with a fine-angled curette, a motorized 2-mm or 2.9-mm shaver, and a 2.9-mm burr until all fibrotic tissue and sclerotic bone are removed. If there is previous screw fixation, the loose screw should be removed to facilitate radical debridement. Any intact cartilage or pseudocapsule around the fracture site should be preserved for better graft containment (Video 2). Both ends of the nonunion are burred until

cancellous bone with or without punctate bleeding is reached (**Fig. 7**) and confirmed by viewing at the MCR portal. A tourniquet is not necessary and, therefore, vascularity of the remaining bone fragments can be accurately assessed. Further curettage of the proximal fragment can be performed through the STT portal if necessary (see **Fig. 5**). If bone bleeding is not obvious or is uncertain, stop the saline irrigation temporarily to reduce the hydrostatic pressure inside the joint and observe for any trivial bleeding.

Correction of Scaphoid Deformity

After adequate debridement and curettage, the 2 fragments of the nonunion should be mobile enough for subsequent reduction. Any humpback and DISI (dorsal intercalated segment instability) deformity should be identified and corrected by the following:

1. Using the Linscheid maneuver. In the presence of an intact scapholunate (SL) ligament, extension deformity of the proximal pole of scaphoid is corrected by bending the wrist to realign the extended lunate with the radius (ie, to restore the normal radiolunate [RL] angle). The RL joint is then temporarily transfixed with a percutaneous 1.6-mm K-wire inserted from dorsal distal radius through a small stab wound (**Fig. 8**). To avoid the risk of entrapping the extensor tendons, an oscillating mode of the K-wire driver should be used.
2. By grasping and traction on the patient's thumb and thenar area (**Fig. 9**) with a surgical towel placed underneath the operated forearm, to ulnar deviate, supinate, and extend the wrist to realign the distal scaphoid fragment with the

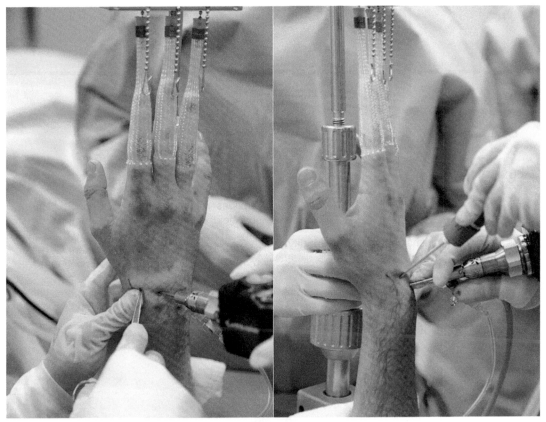

Fig. 5. An arthroscopic burr was inserted through the STT portal for more direct tackling of the nonunion site.

proximal scaphoid fragment. This maneuver favors restoration of the normal scaphoid length and alignment.

3. By inserting a 1.6-mm K-wire into to the distal fragment as a joystick manipulation, especially in distal-third nonunion.

4. Using a probe to manipulate the fragment within the MCJt.

Once the fracture fragments are well aligned, they are transfixed with a 1.1-mm K-wire inserted percutaneously from the scaphoid tubercle under

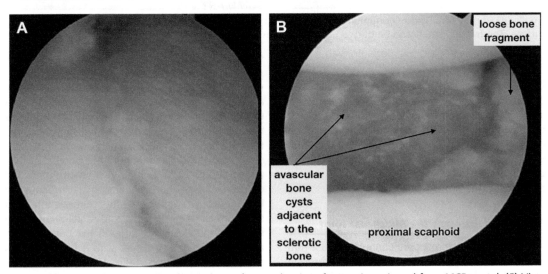

Fig. 6. (*A*) Cleavage line in scaphoid articular surface at the site of nonunion, viewed from MCR portal. (*B*) View from MCU portal. Frank fracture nonunion gap was found with cysts and loose fracture fragment.

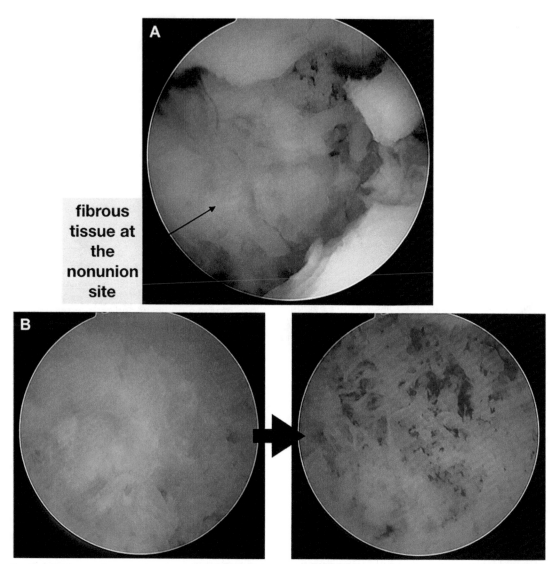

fibrous tissue at the nonunion site

Fig. 7. (*A*) Fibrous tissue at the nonunion site has to be removed. (*B*) Arthroscopic image of a nonunion fracture surface. The fracture site has to be burred until cancellous bone trabeculae are seen.

fluoroscopic guidance (see **Fig. 9**). The K-wire should aim eccentrically at a more radial and proximal location across the nonunion site so that the pin would not block the placement and impaction of the bone graft inserted from the MCJt (**Fig. 10**). When the fixation is complete, the hand can be put back to the traction tower for bone grafting procedure.

Bone Graft Through the Midcarpal Joint

Another, bigger arthroscopic cannula (eg, 3.2 mm or 4.5 mm for bigger wrist) is introduced through an appropriate portal directly opposing the fracture defect. For fractures located at the proximal two-thirds of the scaphoid, the MCR portal is the most direct. For distal-third fractures, an STT portal can be considered. Cancellous bone graft is harvested from the iliac crest using either a trephine or an open technique through a small incision (**Fig. 11**). The volume of the bone graft obtained should be at least 3 to 5 times that of the defect because the graft has to be impacted in the defect to increase its compaction and strength. Bone graft is cut into small chips using scissors and delivered through the cannula with a slightly undersized trocar with a flat end, such as a bone biopsy trocar (**Fig. 12**). The arm tourniquet can be inflated to enhance visibility during the graft impaction process.

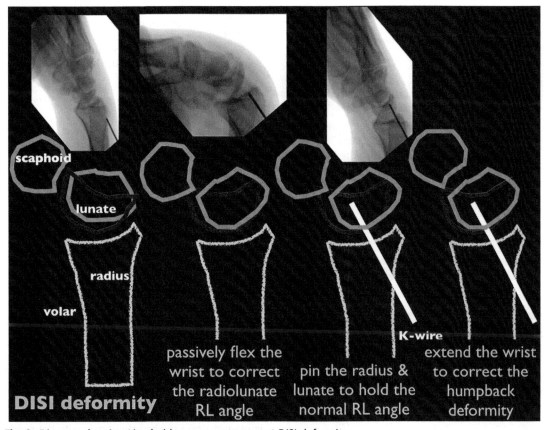

scaphoid

lunate

radius

volar

DISI deformity

passively flex the wrist to correct the radiolunate RL angle

pin the radius & lunate to hold the normal RL angle

K-wire

extend the wrist to correct the humpback deformity

Fig. 8. Diagram showing Linscheid maneuver to correct DISI deformity.

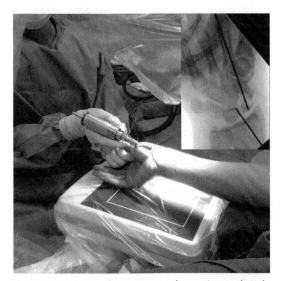

Fig. 9. Grasping and traction on the patient's thumb, with a surgical towel placed underneath the operated forearm, to ulnar deviate and extend the wrist to realign the distal scaphoid fragment with the proximal scaphoid fragment. A K-wire was inserted from the scaphoid tuberosity to the proximal fragment.

The most proximal and dorsal part of the defect has to be filled up first to avoid subsequent graft void. Empty space previously occupied by a loose screw should also be filled in first.

In very proximal fractures, the nonunion site can be directly communicating with the RCJt. To avoid spillage of bone graft from the MCJt into the RCJt, a pediatric size 6 urinary catheter is inserted into the RCJt through the 3-4 portal and insufflated with saline, providing a mechanical block from the bone graft going into the RCJt (**Fig. 13**, Videos 3 and 4).

A small depressor, as shown in **Fig. 14**, is used at intervals to impact the bone graft into the fracture gap and mould to the shape of the articular surface of scaphoid (Video 5). Confirm the completeness and adequacy of the graft filling by fluoroscopy. After completion of impaction bone grafting, the MCJt and RCJt are inspected to remove any spilled out bone graft debris. MCJt is aspirated dry and 1 mL of fibrin glue is applied on the surface of the graft substance (**Fig. 15**). Traction is released to allow the natural compression from the capitate onto the graft.

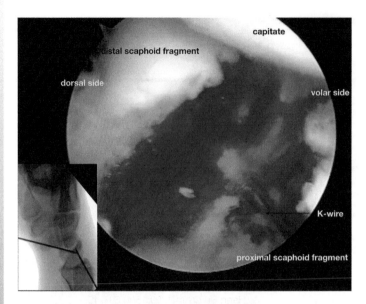

Fig. 10. View from MCU portal. The pin should be situated in a volar and proximal position at the nonunion site so that subsequent bone grafting is not blocked by the K-wire.

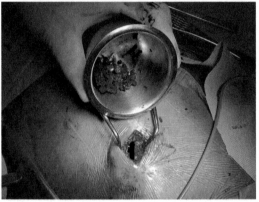
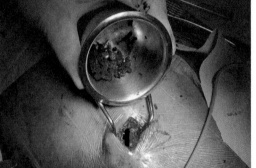

Fig. 11. The left iliac crest is used as a bone graft donor site. The amount of bone graft should be about 3 times that of the nonunion defect.

Fracture Fixation

Percutaneous screw fixation
Percutaneous screw fixation is indicated when the bone defect is small, and located at the middle-third of the scaphoid, with sizeable proximal and distal fragments (Fig. 16). A screw guide pin is placed along the scaphoid axis with the surgical techniques described elsewhere.[57,58] Cannulated screw is used but excessive compression should be avoided to prevent graft extrusion and collapse of the nonunion site. After screw fixation, the initial transfixing 1.1-mm K-wire is then removed.

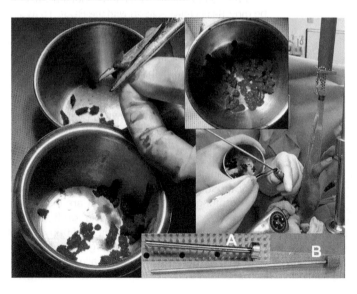

Fig. 12. Bone graft was cut into small pieces (right, left, and inset) and delivered to the nonunion site through (A) a trocar cannula with no side hole and impacted with (B) a trocar with flat tip and of smaller diameter than the trocar cannula.

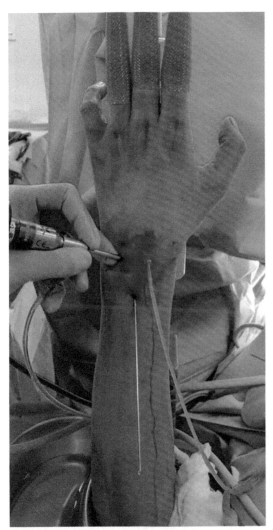

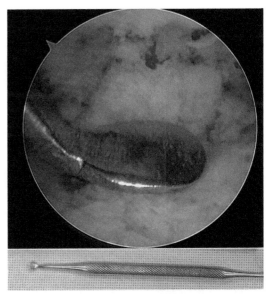

Fig. 14. Bone graft (*top*) was impacted and contoured by a depressor (*bottom*).

Percutaneous multiple Kirschner wire fixation

Percutaneous multiple Kirschner wire fixation is indicated when the bone defect is sizable, particularly in proximal or distal-third nonunion, and for nonunion with previous screw fixation (**Fig. 17**). It is difficult to achieve an ideal position while having sufficient bone purchase when using a screw in these situations. This risks bone fragmentation, especially the proximal pole; the screw cutting out; excessive compression causing recurrence of humpback deformity; and graft extrusion. Two or 3 additional 1.1-mm K-wires are inserted adjacent to the initial transfixing K-wire. SL or scaphocapitate K-wire can also be used for an unstable nonunion. The K-wires are cut short and buried under the skin and removed 10 to 12 weeks later.

Fig. 13. For proximal scaphoid fracture that communicated with the RCJt, a Foley catheter was inserted through the 3-4 portal and was insufflated to block the bone graft going into the RCJt.

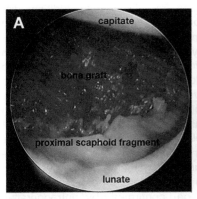

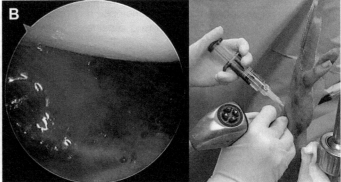

Fig. 15. Fibrin glue was applied through MCR portal to cover the bone graft (*left*). (*A*) Before tissue glue application. (*B*) After tissue glue application.

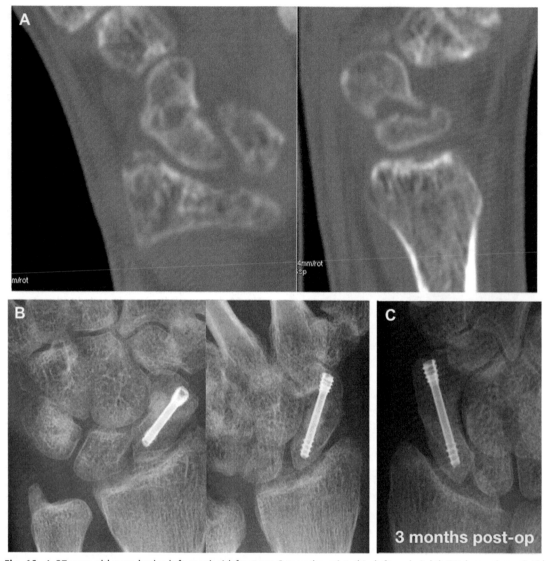

Fig. 16. A 27-year-old man had a left scaphoid fracture 6 months prior. (*A: left* and *right*) CT showed scaphoid nonunion. (*B*) He was treated with ABG and percutaneous screw. (*C*) There was complete union at 3 months and he was asymptomatic with good function. Post-op, postoperative

The wounds are opposed with steristrips. If there is an RL K-wire, it is left exposed outside the skin for early removal.

SPECIAL CONDITIONS
Early Scaphoid Nonunion Advanced Collapse Wrist

Early SNAC changes involving the radial styloid and distal scaphoid fragment is not a contraindication for ABG, provided that an adequate radial styloidectomy is done to reduce the subsequent impingement (**Fig. 18**). Arthroscopic radial styloidectomy gives better visualization and, therefore, preserves the important stabilizing structure of

radioscaphocapitate ligament. An arthroscope is passed through the 4-5 portal toward the dorsal aspect of the radial styloid. A 2.9-mm burr is introduced from the 3-4 portal, and burrs on the arthritic styloid to create a 5-mm depth defect until an even, smooth surface is obtained. Caution should be exercised to prevent burring too far into the scaphoid fossa. The volar aspect of radial styloid should be spared because it is the important origin of the radioscaphocapitate ligament and impingement symptoms seldom arise from this area. Adequacy of radial styloidectomy can be confirmed by intraoperative fluoroscopy.

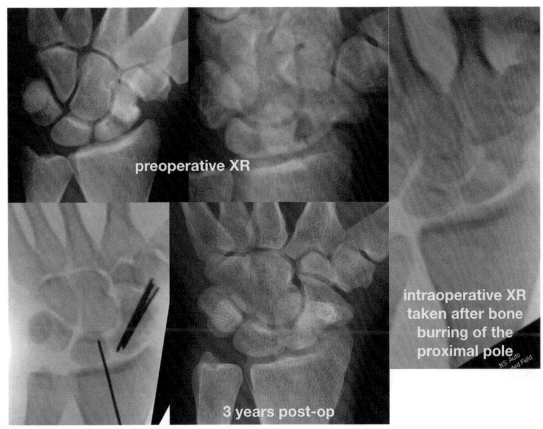

preoperative XR

intraoperative XR taken after bone burring of the proximal pole

3 years post-op

Fig. 17. A 17-year-old student with right scaphoid fracture 3.5 months prior. ABG was done and fixed with 3 K-wires across the fracture site and he was asymptomatic with good function. XR, radiograph.

POSTOPERATIVE CARE

A short arm plaster slab is provided and maintained for 2 weeks. In cases with DISI deformity, the transfixing pin across the RL joint is removed by 2 weeks. A wrist brace is then fabricated. If the nonunion site is stable, active wrist mobilization out of the brace under supervision of a hand therapist is initiated at 2 weeks. A radiograph is taken at regular intervals to monitor the progress of graft incorporation and bone healing. Once clinical and radiological union is confirmed, the K-wires can be removed under local anesthesia, typically at 10 to 12 weeks postoperatively. Passive wrist mobilization is initiated once union is established. Hand and upper limb strengthening can follow, usually at 12 to 16 weeks postoperatively.

RESULTS

From April 1997 to December 2016, 125 ABGs were done for 111 established symptomatic nonunions and 14 delayed union cases on 117 men

and 8 women, with an average age of 28 years (range 14–66 years). Nonunion was defined as no radiological feature of healing at least 12 weeks postinjury, whereas delayed union was defined as poor radiological sign of healing in fractures less than 12 weeks postinjury with fracture site bony resorption, with or without adjacent sclerosis or cyst formation. All patients presented with wrist pain, stiffness, and disturbance to their daily activities and works. Dominant hands were involved in 68 cases (54%), 41 patients (33%) were chronic smokers, and 58 were heavy manual workers. Sixty percent were sports-related injuries. The median duration of pathologic injury was 42 months (range 1–480 months). There were 16 distal-third, 67 middle-third, and 42 proximal-third scaphoid fractures; and there were 8 proximal pole fractures. Twelve patients had received previous surgeries for scaphoid fracture or nonunion but the fracture had still not united. There were 17 cases of proximal pole avascular necrosis as shown in contrast MRI (**Fig. 19**). DISI deformity was found in 60 wrists (48%), in which 13 were distal-third fracture, 30 middle-

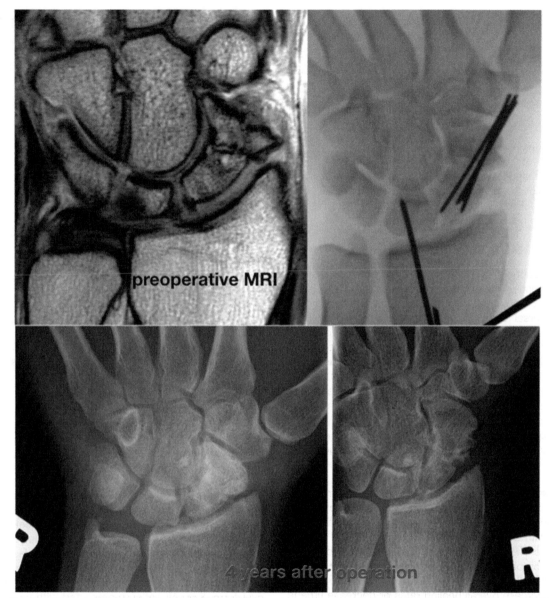

Fig. 18. 27-year-old life guard with right scaphoid fracture 10 years prior. He had persistent wrist pain. MRI showed SNAC1 wrist changes (*A, upper left*). Arthroscopy also showed thinned cartilage at proximal aspect of capitate. Radial styloidectomy and ABG were done (*B, upper right*). He enjoyed a pain-free wrist with better strength (grip power 56 kg) till the last follow-up 4 years after the operation. His wrist range of motion was the same as preoperatively. (*C, lower left and right*) showed the XRs 4 years after the operation.

third, and 17 proximal-third (2 were proximal pole). Radiological stage I or II SNAC wrist changes were found in 24 wrists.

All patients were assessed by occupational therapists before and during the operation, and at the final follow-up. The range of wrist motion, grip power, wrist function performance score, pain score, and return to work status were charted. The wrist functional performance score developed by the authors' hospital was modeled on the findings of D.L. Nelson.[59] It consists of 10 common standardized tasks of activities of daily living (ADL) performed by the patient under the scrutiny of an occupational therapist (**Fig. 20**). The performance on each task was rated by the therapist according to a 4-point scale, giving a maximum total of 40 for a normal performance. A pain score on a 3-point scale

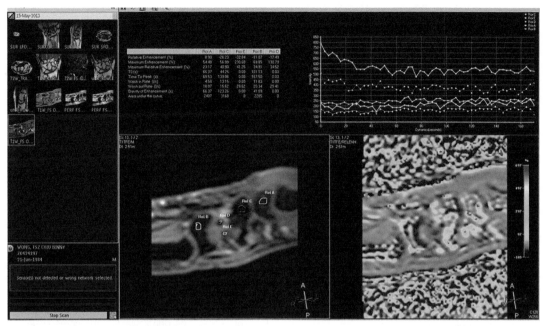

Fig. 19. Contrast vascular flow MRI study showed poor vascularity of proximal scaphoid fragment.

was rated by the patient according to the pain level perceived during the performance of each ADL task, with the total score ranging from 0 to 20.

Postoperative radiographs and computed tomography (CT) scans were used at intervals to monitor bony union, degenerative changes, and alignment of scaphoid, including SL angle and anteroposterior (AP) intrascaphoid angle.

All cases were completed arthroscopically. The mean operation duration was 213 minutes (range 90–420 minutes). Twenty-five patients had concomitant procedures, including arthroscopic-assisted reduction of distal radius fracture and internal fixation (3), thumb tendon transfer (1), thumb metacarpophalangeal joint (MCPJ) fusion (1), thumb MCPJ arthroscopic arthrolysis (1), arthroscopic curettage and bone grafting of lunate bone cyst (1), distal phalanx fracture nonunion bone grafting and internal fixation (1), arthroscopic radial styloidectomy (10), arthroscopic Wafer procedure (1), SL ligament thermal shrinkage and pinning (2), arthroscopic-assisted SL ligament repair (1), and triangular fibrocartilage complex (TFCC) debridement (4). We used cannulated screws in 38 cases and multiple K-wires for 87 cases for scaphoid fixation. One patient lost follow-up at 3 weeks after surgery. The average follow-up duration was 34 months (range 3–125 months). Overall union rate was 90.3% (112 out of 124). The average radiological union time was 14 weeks (range 6–80 weeks). Poor intraoperative vascularity might have predisposed to persistent

nonunion but did not preclude union entirely. Poor proximal fragment bleeding was found in 33 cases, whereas it was fair in 26 cases. Correlation of union status and vascularity of proximal scaphoid fragment is shown in **Table 1**. Poor intraoperative bleeding of proximal scaphoid still permitted union in 27 out of 33 cases (81.8%), whereas good bleeding predicted union in 62 out of 65 cases (95.4%).

At final clinical follow-up, there was no pain on exertion or forceful loading in 67 patients (54%), whereas exertion on a visual analog scale (VAS) in the remaining 57 patients improved from an average of 5 (range 0–9) to 1.7 (range 0–7). There was improvement in the ADL performance score from an average of 34.2 to 38.6 and in the ADL pain score from an average of 4.7 to 1.3, and grip power improved from an average of 28.2 kg to 36.2 kg. There was no change in wrist range in extension, radial deviation, and ulnar deviation; however, the flexion range was mildly decreased from average 58.2° to 55.8°. All patients had inconspicuous scars (**Fig. 21**). The final SL angle was 60.9° (49°–76°) and the average AP intrascaphoid angle was 32.6° (19°–40°).

Three patients developed pin tract infections. In all 3 cases, K-wires were left protruded outside the skin. One was due to pseudomonas and required K-wire removal prematurely at 5 weeks. The other 2 were caused by *Staphylococcus* and the infection was well controlled with antibiotics and pin tract dressing. Bone union was not affected.

Prince of Wales Hospital
Occupational Therapy Department
Assessment of ADL Performance for Wrist Injury

Date					
Post-op (weeks)					
ADL Tasks by Affected Side		Performance	Pain	Performance	Pain
Wash back	(F,N,S,Rd,Ud,Pi)				
Pull out drawer 7lbs	(N,S,Gr)				
Pour out water from full pot	(N,F,Ud)				
Turn door knob/ turn key	(N,P,S)				
Open gate	(E,S)				
Lift weight 5lbs	(N,E,Ud,Gr)				
Write name	(E,Ud,Pi)				
Wring towel dry	(P,S,Gr,Ud,Rd,E,F)				
Hold a wok	(E,Ud,Gr,S)				
Open jar lid	(N,Ud,Rd,Gr)				
Total Performance Score		/ 40		/ 40	
Total Pain Score		/ 20		/ 20	
Remarks					
Overall Comment					
Wrist range		L	R	L	R
Extension					
Flexion					
Radial Deviation					
Ulnar Deviation					
Pronation					
Supination					
VAS Pain on Exertion					
Power Grip (kg)					
Lateral Pinch (kg)					

Performance
4: can do without difficulty and pain free
3: can do with minimum difficulty or pain, but with satisfactory outcome
2: can do with some modification of activities, with awkward and pain
1: pain affect the performance and the quality is poor, would stop doing it most of the time
0: cannot do at all
Pain
2: pain free in doing
1: tolerated pain in doing
0: intolerable pain in doing

Wrist/ forearm position
E   Extension
F   Flexion
S   Supination
P   Pronation
Ud   Ulnar deviation
Rd   Radial deviation
Gr   Gripping action
Pi   Pinching action
N   Neutral wrist

Fig. 20. The wrist function assessment data sheet to be performed by an occupational therapist. It consists of 5 elements: performance evaluation, pain evaluation, wrist range of motion, verbal analog pain scale, and grip and pinch strength.

Table 1
Correlation of union status and vascularity of proximal scaphoid fragment

Number of Patients in Different Degree of Vascularity of Proximal Fragment			Final Union Status after ABG (Number of Patients)
Good	Fair	Poor	
62	23	27	Union (112)
1	1	4	Fibrous union (6)
2	2	2	Nonunion (6)
Total: 65	Total: 26	Total: 33	—

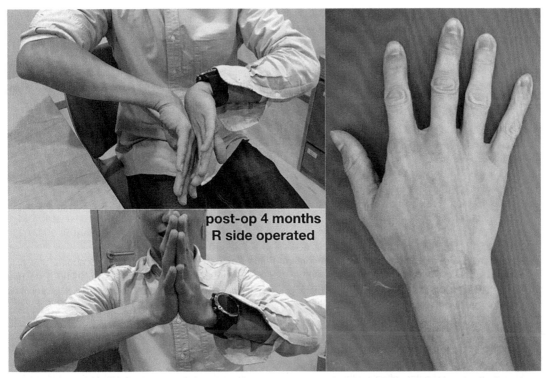

Fig. 21. Right wrist ABG done 4 months prior. The scars were inconspicuous. (*upper left*) wrist flexion range, (*lower left*) wrist extension range, 4 months after the operation. (*Lower, right*) the scars were inconspicuous.

Because of these complications in our early series, all K-wires were buried underneath the skin in subsequent ABG operations for later removal. There was no more pin tract infection but 6 cases of K-wire loosening and protrusion outside skin caused irritation. There were 2 cases of donor site hematoma at the iliac crest and 1 case of lateral cutaneous nerve of thigh neurapraxia. All symptoms resolved spontaneously and completely. Two patients experienced reflex sympathetic dystrophy in which 1 subsided spontaneously and another had arthroscopic arthrolysis 1 year after the operation to improve wrist range.

There were 6 persistent nonunion requiring revision surgeries. One required revision grafting with vascularized distal radius bone graft. In another case, because of severe scaphoid collapse, scapholunate-capitate fusion was done, augmented with a vascularized distal radius bone graft. One patient was salvaged with radioscapholunate fusion augmented with vascularized distal radius bone graft. Three patients received revision ABG and finally got union at 10 weeks, 10 weeks, and 12 months, respectively. There was 1 case with proximal pole resorption but this was clinically asymptomatic. One patient with progressive SNAC wrist changes refused further surgery although pain persisted at a level of 6 on a 10-point VAS scale.

SUPPLEMENTARY DATA

Supplementary data related to this article can be found online at https://doi.org/10.1016/j.hcl.2019.03.003.

REFERENCES

1. Ruby LK, Leslie BM. Wrist arthritis associated with scaphoid nonunion. Hand Clin 1987;3(4): 529–39.
2. Ruby LK, Stinson J, Belsky MR. The natural history of scaphoid nonunion: a review of 55 cases. J Bone Joint Surg Am 1985;67:428–32.
3. Mack GR, Bosse MJ, Gelberman RH, et al. The natural history of scaphoid non-union. J Bone Joint Surg Am 1984;66:504–9.
4. Vender MI, Watson HK, Wiener BD, et al. Degenerative change in symptomatic scaphoid nonunion. J Hand Surg Am 1987;12:514–9.
5. Inoue G, Sakuma M. The natural history of scaphoid nonunion: radiographical and clinical analysis in 102 cases. Arch Orthop Trauma Surg 1996;115:1–4.
6. Gehrmann S, Roeger T, Kaufmann R, et al. Wrist motion analysis in scaphoid nonunion. Eur J Trauma Emerg Surg 2016;42(1):11–4.
7. Matti H. Technik und Resultate meiner pseudarthrosenoperation. Zentralbl Chir 1936;63:1442–53.

8. Matti H. Über die Behandlung der Navicularefraktur und der Refraktura patellae durch Plombierung mit Spongiosa. Zentralbl Chir 1937;64(41):2353–9.

9. Russe O. Fracture of the carpal navicular. Diagnosis, non-operative treatment and operative treatment. J Bone Joint Surg Am 1960;42-A:759–68.

10. Fisk GR. Carpal instability and the fractured scaphoid. Ann R Coll Surg Engl 1970;46:63.

11. Fernandez DL. A technique for anterior wedge-shaped grafts for scaphoid nonunions with carpal instability. J Hand Surg Am 1984;9(5):733–7.

12. Maruthainar N, Rasquinha VJ, Gallagher P. The treatment of scaphoid nonunion: A review of a novel technique using precision bone grafting compared with Herbert screw fixation and bone graft. J Hand Surg Br 2000;25(5):427–30.

13. Leung YF, Ip SPS, Cheuk C, et al. Trephine bone grafting technique for the treatment of scaphoid nonunion. J Hand Surg Am 2001;26(5):893–900.

14. Pinder RM, Brkljac M, Rix L, et al. Treatment of scaphoid nonunion: a systemic review of existing evidence. J Hand Surg Am 2015;40(9):1791–805.

15. Merrell GA, Wolfe SW, Slade JF 3rd. Treatment of scaphoid nonunions: quantitative meta-analysis of the literature. J Hand Surg Am 2002;27(4):685–91.

16. Shah J, Jones WA. Factors affecting the outcome in 50 cases of scaphoid nonunion treated with Herbert screw fixation. J Hand Surg Br 1998;23:680–5.

17. Alluri R, Yin C, Iorio M, et al. A critical appraisal of vascularized bone grafting for scaphoid nonunion. J Wrist Surg 2017;6(3):251–7.

18. Judet R, Roy-Camille R, Guillamn JL. Traitement de pseudoarthrose du scaphoid carpien par le greffon pedicule. Revue de Chirurgie Orthopédique 1972; 58:699–705.

19. Braun RM. Pronator pedicle bone grafting in the forearm and proximal carpal row. J Hand Surg 1983;8:612–3.

20. Kuhlmann JN, Guerin-Surville H, Mimoun M, et al. Greffon osseux pedicule d'aide vasculaire au niveau du poignet. Acta Orthop Belg 1986;52:753–70.

21. Kuhlmann JN, Mimoun M, Boabighi A, et al. Vascularized bone graft pedicled on the volar carpal artery for non-union of the scaphoid. J Hand Surg Br 1987; 12(2):203–10.

22. Guimberteau JC, Panconi B. Recalcitrant non-union of the scaphoid treated with a vascularised bone graft based on the ulnar artery. J Bone Joint Surg Am 1990;72(1):88–97.

23. Zaidemberg C, Siebert JW, Angrigiani C. A new vascularized bone graft for scaphoid nonunion. J Hand Surg Am 1991;16(3):474–8.

24. Brunelli F, Brunelli G, Nanfito F. An anatomical study of the vascularisation of the first dorsal interosseous space in the hand, and a description of a bony pedicle graft arising from the second metacarpal bone. Surg Radiol Anat 1991;13(1):73–5.

25. Mathoulin C, Brunelli F. Further experience with the index metacarpal vascularized bone graft. J Hand Surg Br 1998;23:311–7.

26. Yuceturk A, Isiklar ZU, Tuncay C, et al. Treatment of scaphoid nonunions with a vascularised bone graft based on the first dorsal metacarpal artery. J Hand Surg Br 1997;22:425–7.

27. Pechlaner S, Hussl H, Kunzel KH. Alternative surgical method in pseudarthroses of the scaphoid bone. Prospective study. Handchir Mikrochir Plast Chir 1987;19:302–5.

28. Doi K, Oda T, Soo-Heong T, et al. Free vascularized bone graft for nonunion of the scaphoid. J Hand Surg Am 2000;25(3):507–19.

29. Veitch S, Blake SM, David H. Proximal scaphoid rib graft arthroplasty. J Bone Joint Surg Br 2007;89(2): 196–201.

30. Straw RG, Davis TR, Dias JJ. Scaphoid nonunion: treatment with a pedicled vascularized bone graft based on the 1,2 intercompartmental supraretinacular branch of the radial artery. J Hand Surg Br 2002; 27:413.

31. Boyer MI, von Schroeder HP, Axelrod TS. Scaphoid nonunion with avascular necrosis of the proximal pole. Treatment with a vascularized bone graft from the dorsum of the distal radius. J Hand Surg Br 1998;23:686–90.

32. Chang MA, Bishop AT, Berger RA. The outcomes and complications of 1,2-intercompartmental supraretinacular artery pedicled vascularized bone grafting of scaphoid nonunions. J Hand Surg Am 2006; 31:387–96.

33. Alluri R, Yin C, Iorio M, et al. Vascularized bone grafting in scaphoid nonunion. Hand 2017;12(2):127–34.

34. Rajagopalan BM, Squire DS, Samuels LO. Results of Herbert screw fixation with bone grafting for the treatment of nonunion of the scaphoid. J Bone Joint Surg Am 1999;81(1):48–52.

35. Sawaizumi T, Nanno M, Nanbu A, et al. Vascularised bone graft from base of the second metacarpal for refractory nonunion of the scaphoid. J Bone Joint Surg Br 2004;86:1007–12.

36. Tsai TT, Chao EK, Tu YK, et al. Management of Scaphoid nonunion with avascular necrosis using 1, 2 intercompartmental supraretinacular arterial bone grafts. Chang Gung Med J 2002;25:321–8.

37. Segalman KA, Graham TJ. Scaphoid proximal pole fractures and nonunions. J Am Soc Surg Hand 2004;4:233–49.

38. Dehghani M, Soltanmohamadi M, Tahririan MA, et al. Management of scaphoid nonunion with avascular necrosis using 1,2 intercompartmental supraretinacular arterial bone graft. Adv Biomed Res 2014;3:185.

39. Ditsios K, Konstantinidis I, Agas K, et al. Comparative meta-analysis on the various vascularised bone flaps used for treatment of scaphoid nonunion. J Orthop Res 2017;35(5):1076–85.

40. Vedung T, Vinnars B. Ectopic bone formation after medial femoral condyle graft to scaphoid nonunion. J Wrist Surg 2014;3(1):46–9.

41. Werdin F, Jaminet P, Naegele B, et al. Reconstruction of scaphoid nonunion fractures of the proximal one third with a vascularized bone graft from the distal radius. Eplasty 2014;14:E24.

42. Slade JF III, Dodds SD. Minimally invasive management of scaphoid nonunions. Clin Orthop Relat Res 2006;445:108–19.

43. Slade JF III, Gillen T. Retrospective review of 234 scaphoid fractures and nonunions treated with arthroscopy for union and complications. Scand J Surg 2008;97:280–9.

44. Smith DK, An KN, Cooney WP III, et al. Effects of a scaphoid waist osteotomy on carpa kinematics. J Orthop Res 1989;7:590–8.

45. Kamal RN, Starr A, Akelman E. Carpal kinematics and kinetics. J Hand Surg Am 2016;41(10):1011–8.

46. Munk PL, Lee MJ, Logan PM, et al. Scaphoid bone waist fractures, acute and chronic: imaging with different techniques. AJR Am J Roentgenol 1997;168:779–86.

47. Marai GE, Crisco JJ, Laidlaw DH. A kinematics-based method for generating cartilage maps and deformations in the multi-articulating wrist joint from CT images. Conf Proc IEEE Eng Med Biol Soc 2006;1:2079–82.

48. Dwek JR. The periosteum: what is it, where is it, and what mimics it in its absence? Skeletal Radiol 2010;39:319–23.

49. Demirag B, Sarisozen B, Ozer O, et al. Enhancement of tendon-bone healing of anterior cruciate ligament grafts by blockade of matrix metalloproteinases. J Bone Joint Surg Am 2005;87(11):2401–10.

50. Abedi G, Alizadeh R, Biabangardi B, et al. Effect of synovial fluid on intercondylar fracture in cats. Ann Bio Res 2013;4(9):87–91.

51. Berg EE, Pollard ME, Kang Q. Interarticular bone tunnel healing. Arthroscopy 2001;17:189–95.

52. Hazelton RA, Vedam R, Masci PP, et al. Partial purification and characterisation of a synovial fluid inhibitor of osteoblasts. Ann Rheum Dis 1990;49:121–4.

53. Gelberman RH, Gross MS. The vascularity of the wrist. Identification of arterial patterns at risk. Clin Orthop Relat Res 1986;202:40–9.

54. Handley RC, Pooley J. The venous anatomy of the scaphoid. J Anat 1991;178:115–8.

55. Barton NJ. Twenty questions about scaphoid fractures. J Hand Surg Br 1992;17:289–310.

56. Ong TYM, Ho PC, Wong WYC, et al. Wrist arthroscopy under portal site local anaesthesia (PSLA) without tourniquet. J Wrist Surg 2012;1(2):149–52.

57. Wong WYC, Ho PC. Minimal invasive management of scaphoid fractures: from fresh to nonunion. Hand Clin 2011;27(3):291–307.

58. Ho PC, Wong WYC, Tse WL. Arthroscopic bone grafting for scaphoid nonunion. Chapter 35. In: Buijze GA, Jupiter JB, editors. Scaphoid fractures: evidence-based management. St. Louis (MO): Elsevier; 2018. p. 320–54.

59. Nelson DL. Function wrist motion. Hand Clin 1997;13(1):83–92.

The Role of Vascularized Bone Grafting in Scaphoid Nonunion

Nicole M. Sgromolo, MD[a], Peter C. Rhee, DO, MS[b],*

KEYWORDS

- Scaphoid nonunion • Proximal pole avascular necrosis • Vascularized bone graft
- Nonvascularized bone graft • Humpback deformity

KEY POINTS

- Diagnosis of avascular necrosis should involve intraoperative evaluation of scaphoid vascularity following tourniquet deflation.
- In the setting of avascular necrosis, vascularized bone graft should be used to restore blood flow and promote osseous healing.
- The appropriate vascularized bone graft to be used for scaphoid reconstruction is determined by the presence of a preoperative scaphoid flexion (humpback) deformity or carpal collapse.

INTRODUCTION

The scaphoid is the most commonly fractured bone within the carpus, accounting for 70% of all carpal injuries. However, despite being relatively common, these fractures remain challenging to treat.[1,2] Mostly covered by articular cartilage, the scaphoid derives its blood supply mainly through retrograde flow from the dorsal scaphoid branch of the radial artery.[3] As a result, these fractures remain at an elevated risk of nonunion and avascular necrosis (AVN).[3] AVN occurs predominantly in fractures affecting the proximal third of the scaphoid.[4,5]

The risk of nonunion following fracture of the scaphoid varies and has been reported to occur in approximately 10% to 12% of cases.[2,6] This number may be as high as 55% in those patients with initial displacement greater than 1 mm.[7–9] Additional factors placing patients at risk for nonunion include delay in treatment, coexisting carpal instability, and localization of the fracture to the proximal pole.[2]

Nonunion is defined as an absence of bony healing persisting 6 months or longer following the injury or surgery.[10] Nonunion is diagnosed with the use of plain radiography or advanced imaging, and is evident as a persistent fracture line with associated progressive sclerosis, bone resorption, and cyst formation.[11,12] Due to the importance of scaphoids in carpal mechanics, longstanding nonunion leads to predictable changes, including carpal instability, so-called humpback deformity, scaphoid collapse, and a progressive pattern of carpal arthritis referred to as scaphoid nonunion advanced collapse arthritis.[6,13,14]

MANAGEMENT PRINCIPLES FOR SCAPHOID RECONSTRUCTION

The goals of treatment following scaphoid nonunion include achieving bony union, correcting deformity, achieving reduction of pain, and preventing further degenerative changes.[15] For successful treatment of scaphoid nonunions, rigid fixation is necessary, which can be achieved with

Disclosure Statement: None.

[a] Department of Orthopaedic Surgery, Brooke Army Medical Center, Fort Sam Houston, San Antonio, TX, USA;
[b] Department of Orthopedic Surgery, Mayo Clinic, 200 First Street Southwest, Rochester, MN 55905, USA
* Corresponding author.
E-mail address: rhee.peter@mayo.edu

Hand Clin 35 (2019) 315–322
https://doi.org/10.1016/j.hcl.2019.03.004

hand.theclinics.com

headless compression screws (HCSs), Kirschner (K)-wires, plates, or staples. In those patients with preserved carpal stability, normal scaphoid alignment, minimal bone loss, and intact proximal pole vascularity, defined as intraoperative bleeding after tourniquet takedown (**Fig. 1**), rigid fixation alone may be sufficient to achieve bony union.[16–18] This is predicated on obtaining adequate fixation in the proximal and distal fracture fragments to provide structural support.

If the scaphoid is markedly foreshortened, rotated, and/or flexed with a humpback deformity, structural bone graft should be used to correct carpal and scaphoid alignment. Amadio and colleagues[19] noted that in scaphoid malunions with a humpback deformity (lateral intrascaphoid angle ≥45°), satisfactory clinical outcomes accounting for pain, motion, function, and strength were achieved in only 27% (7 of 26) of cases and posttraumatic arthritis developed in 54% (14 of 26) of wrists. This highlights the importance of restoring normal scaphoid geometry and carpal alignment to increase the rate of union but also to improve functional outcomes.

The type of bone graft used to restore scaphoid anatomy has been a frequent area of debate. Although the site of nonvascularized bone graft harvest likely does not influence union rates, a large meta-analysis from Merrell and colleagues[20] in 2002 suggested that vascularized bone graft (VBG) was beneficial in cases of AVN. The specific type of VBG used to reconstruct a scaphoid nonunion with proximal pole AVN is dictated by the absence or presence of a humpback deformity or carpal collapse.[20–22] However, questions remain regarding the indications and true benefits of VBGs for scaphoid nonunions. This article is devoted to determining the indications for VBG for scaphoid nonunion.

THE ROLE OF NONVASCULARIZED BONE GRAFTING

Nonvascularized autogenous bone grafting has traditionally been used in the treatment of most scaphoid nonunions.[23–26] In 1960, Otto Russe[23] first described the use of a nonvascularized iliac crest bone graft in the treatment of scaphoid nonunions, yielding a 91% union rate with bony healing occurring in 21 of 22 subjects. When first combined with rigid fixation (2.7-mm cortical screw), Fernandez[24] demonstrated a high success rate with 19 of 20 scaphoid nonunions healing following nonvascularized iliac crest bone grafting at an average of 9.8 weeks. This set the precedent for managing scaphoid nonunions with a combination of rigid fixation and autogenous nonvascularized bone grafting. Nonvascularized bone graft can be harvested as corticocancellous or cancellous grafts from sites that include the iliac crest, volar or dorsal distal radius, olecranon, or the medial femoral condyle.

Nonvascularized bone grafting is a valid management option in the treatment of scaphoid nonunions without AVN. This method of autogenous bone grafting is advantageous because it is less technically demanding than vascularized bone grafting while still maintaining a high rate of union. Healing occurs by creeping substitution and resorption.[1,27] Though union rates vary throughout the literature, nonvascularized bone grafting seems to be successful in the treatment of scaphoid nonunions.[25,26] Daly and colleagues[26] noted a 96% (25 of 26) union rate at a median of 4 months (range 2–12 months) after

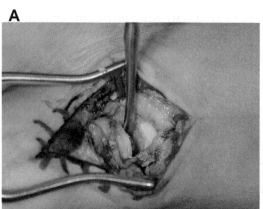
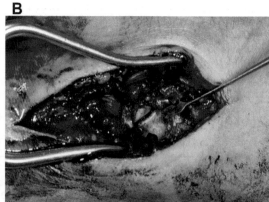

Fig. 1. Intraoperative assessment of proximal pole vascularity in scaphoid nonunions. (*A*) The proximal pole of the scaphoid is examined, with the tourniquet inflated and (*B*) again after tourniquet is let down, for the presence or absence of punctate bleeding, with the latter indicating AVN.

nonvascularized iliac crest bone grafting with an HCS for scaphoid nonunions with humpback deformity without AVN. Yasuda and colleagues[25] demonstrated a union rate of 100% in 28 scaphoid nonunions treated with nonvascularized bone grafting with 6 distal third, 19 middle third, and 3 proximal third nonunions; however, the investigators did not account for the presence or absence of AVN.

In the presence of AVN, nonvascularized bone grafting has demonstrated limited success.[28,29] Robbins and Carter[28] performed Herbert screw fixation and allograft bone graft reconstruction on 17 subjects who were followed for at least 1 year. These 17 subjects had no punctate bleeding of the proximal pole of the scaphoid at the time of surgery and were deemed to have AVN. Of these, only 9 of 17 subjects went on to complete osseous union based on standard radiographs. They observed a fibrous or partial osseous union in 7 of 17 subjects and a persistent nonunion in 1 subject yielding a complete union rate of only 53%.[28] A meta-analysis that included 36 studies with a total of 1827 scaphoid nonunions, noted that successful union was achieved in 94% of cases treated by nonvascularized bone grafting when no evidence of AVN was detected. However, in a subanalysis of 64 subjects with AVN, nonvascularized bone grafting yielded a union rate of only 47% (14 of 30 subjects).[20] This union rate significantly improved to 88% (30 of 34 subjects) when a VBG was used.[20]

Furthermore, Green[29] performed 45 consecutive surgeries for scaphoid nonunion following the Russe technique of proximal and distal pole excavation, corticocancellous nonvascularized bone grafting without internal fixation.[29] The vascularity of the scaphoid was assessed intraoperatively in each case by observing the presence or absence of punctate bleeding of the scaphoid cancellous bone. He deemed vascularity to be good if there were multiple sites of bleeding and the bone had a pink hue. If there were few sites of bleeding, he classified the bone to be of fair or poor vascularity. If there was no bleeding intraoperatively, the proximal pole was judged to be completely avascular. Of his subjects, he noted 26 to have good vascularity, 14 to have fair or poor vascularity, and 5 to be completely avascular, of which 76% (34 of 45) subjects went on to successful union. Green[29] found a strong correlation between union following nonvascularized bone grafting and scaphoid vascularity. Of those with good vascularity, 24 of 26 scaphoid nonunions achieved complete healing. However, in those with fair or poor vascularity, only 71% (10 of 14) united. Even more compelling, Green[29] found

that none of the 5 subjects with a completely avascular proximal pole achieved union over a mean follow-up of 37 months (range 6–77 months) when nonvascularized bone grafting was used.

When examining the literature, one must look carefully at how the investigators define avascularity to judge the effectiveness of nonvascularized grafts. Rancy and colleagues[30] reported on the outcomes of 35 scaphoid nonunions treated with nonvascularized bone grafting and rigid fixation with an HCS. They observed a union rate of 97% (n = 34) with nonvascularized bone grafts. Proximal pole ischemia was noted on 30% (7 of 23) of preoperative MRI on short tau inversion recovery and proton density sequences, yet no proximal pole fragment was deemed avascular. Additionally, intraoperative assessment revealed fair (n = 19) or good (n = 9) vascularity in 85% (n = 33) of subjects, whereas 5 subjects were noted to have poor vascularity.[30] In this study, the investigators stated that poor bleeding intraoperatively equated to AVN, which may be a false assumption. The presence of some bleeding suggests that none of the fractures were truly avascular.[29]

Similarly, tissue from the nonunion site, proximal pole, and distal pole exhibited greater than or equal to 50% necrotic trabeculae in 44% (14 of 32) and greater than or equal to 50% necrotic marrow fat in 12% (4 of 33) of subjects, whereas only 9% (3 of 33) showed no evidence of bone remodeling.[30] Although not clearly stated, tissue specimens from the fibrous nonunion site, proximal and distal poles were sent as 1 sample by 5 fellowship-trained hand surgeons, thus introducing sampling bias. In addition, all samples were obtained with curettage, which is often not possible in truly sclerotic and avascular bone, thus suggesting that true AVN was not present. Additionally, the investigators state that during the 23-month collection period, no VBGs were performed for any of these cases at their institution; this may suggest that a treatment bias was present within their consecutive cohort of 35 subjects.

THE ROLE OF VASCULARIZED BONE GRAFTING

Vascularized bone grafting, though more technically challenging, offers the advantage of preservation and transfer of osteocytes, thereby improving the wound environment for healing.[31] Vascularized bone grafting leads to primary bone healing rather than creeping substitution, thus resulting in more rapid incorporation and bone union.[32–34] Sunagawa and colleagues[35] demonstrated that blood flow rates at the proximal pole was significantly higher in VBGs at 6 weeks when compared with nonvascularized bone grafts in a canine model, suggesting quicker revascularization of previously avascular segments of bone with VBGs. Increased perfusion over time and influx of both osteogenic and angiogenic factors are additional cited benefits of using VBGs in the management of scaphoid nonunions.[35–38]

Al-Jabri and colleagues[39] performed a systematic review of free vascularized bone grafting in which 12 studies, with a total of 245 cases of scaphoid nonunion, were included. Fifty-six subjects underwent a free VBG from the medial femoral condyle and all went on to successful union. The other 188 subjects were treated with iliac crest VBGs with a union rate of 87.7% (165 of 188 subjects). Another systematic review conducted by Pinder and colleagues[40] cited 23 studies that included a total of 521 scaphoid nonunions that underwent vascularized bone grafting with a union rate of 92%, whereas 35 studies with a total of 993 scaphoid nonunions that were treated with nonvascularized bone grafts had a union rate of 88%. A subgroup analysis was performed on 6 series, including 99 scaphoid nonunions with AVN treated with VBGs (10 free medial femoral condyle, 78 pedicle distal radius, 11 iliac crest nonvascularized bone grafts with combined free vascularized periosteal graft) with a combined union rate of 91%. Additionally, Waitayawinyu and colleagues[41] demonstrated a 93.3% union rate in 28 of 30 scaphoid nonunions with proximal pole AVN reconstructed with a pedicled dorsal distal radius VBG. Optimizing fracture-healing biology most likely results in the high union rates seen after scaphoid nonunion reconstruction.[39–43]

VBGs can be categorized into pedicled or free VBGs. Pedicled VBG are advantageous because they are less technically demanding and require a shorter operative time compared with performing a free VBG. However, free VBGs can typically provide a large interposition graft to improve scaphoid length while simultaneously providing vascularized bone.[44] Pedicled VBGs have been described based on the 1,2 intercompartmental supraretinacular artery (ICSRA), the palmar carpal artery, or the first dorsal metacarpal artery. Free VBGs include the iliac crest, based on the deep circumflex iliac artery, and the free medial femoral condyle or medial femoral trochlear VBGs. Both rely on the descending genicular or superomedial genicular artery.

Grafts from the dorsal distal radius, such as the 1,2 ICSRA or 2,3 ICSRA, are largely used as inlay grafts rather than structural wedge grafts.[31,43,45] Though the 1,2 ICSRA has demonstrated great success with scaphoid nonunions, with documented union rates of 100%, Chang and colleagues[45] found that, in the presence of scaphoid nonunion with AVN, the 1,2 ICSRA VBG had a 50% (12 of 24) union rate.[42,43,46] Of the 14 subjects with AVN and humpback deformity, only 50% (n = 7) achieved complete osseous healing.[45] The reason for these poor outcomes most likely relates to the technical difficulty of using a dorsally based graft to restore scaphoid anatomy; pedicle tension or kinking may lead to vascular compromise. Therefore, the 1,2 ICSRA should only be used in cases of scaphoid nonunions with AVN and no humpback deformity or carpal collapse.

In patients with both carpal collapse and AVN of the proximal pole of the scaphoid, correcting carpal malalignment and restoring normal scaphoid geometry remain integral parts of achieving union.[47] In the presence of AVN and carpal collapse, as defined by a revised carpal height ratio less than or equal to 1.52, a lateral intrascaphoid angle greater than or equal to 45°, or a radiolunate angle greater than or equal to 15°, a structural VBG should be used to correct scaphoid geometry and carpal alignment.[31] Volarly based pedicled distal radius VBGs have been used in scaphoid nonunions without AVN with a reported 100% union rate with improvement in overall carpal height and carpal alignment.[31,48–50] Mathoulin and Haerle[50] described the use of a palmar carpal artery–based pedicled VBG in 17 subjects (15 without and 2 with carpal collapse and no assessment of proximal pole vascularity) with union occurring in all subjects at a mean of 60 days. Subsequently, Mathoulin and Haerle[51] observed a 100% union rate in 72 scaphoid nonunions with humpback deformity treated in the same manner. Similarly, Dailiana and colleagues[48] reported a 100% union rate in 9 scaphoid waist nonunions, of which 1 proximal pole exhibited AVN, that were reconstructed with a VBG based off of the palmar carpal artery.

Free VBG from the medial femoral condyle can effectively reconstruct scaphoid nonunions in the setting of AVN, humpback deformity, and carpal collapse. The free medial femoral condyle VBG is used to correct a humpback deformity and dorsal intercalated segment instability, while providing stout vascularized cortical and cancellous bone for scaphoid reconstruction.[4,31] In the setting of scaphoid nonunion, the free medial femoral condyle VBG has been shown in multiple studies to be successful in achieving union.[44,47,52,53] Doi and colleagues[52] noted complete healing in a series of all 10 scaphoid nonunions with AVN when using free medial femoral condyle VBG as a volar inlay graft. In addition, all wrists were noted to have improvements in carpal height index, scapholunate angle, and capitolunate angle.

In a comparison of 1,2 ICSRA to free medial femoral condyle VBGs in the treatment of scaphoid nonunion with AVN and humpback deformity, Jones and colleagues[53] demonstrated complete union and improvement in postoperative carpal alignment in 12 of 12 subjects treated with a free medial femoral condyle VBG, whereas only 4 of 10 subjects went on to union in those subjects treated with the 1,2 ICSRA VBGs. Similarly, Kollitz and colleagues[47] demonstrated healing in 30 of 32 subjects with scaphoid nonunions with carpal collapse and AVN when treated with the free medial femoral condyle VBG. Reconstructed scaphoids also exhibited significant improvement in lateral intrascaphoid angle, scapholunate angle, and radiolunate angle measurements.

The free medial femoral condyle VBG can be efficacious in the management of persistent scaphoid nonunions after a prior failed scaphoid nonunion surgery.[44] Pulos and colleagues[44] reported on 49 previously operated on scaphoid nonunions, of which 36 had prior bone grafting procedures (distal radius nonvascularized bone grafts = 19, iliac crest nonvascularized bone grafts = 9, 1,2 ICSRA VBGs = 2, and allograft bone = 4) that underwent free medial femoral condyle VBG at a mean of 15 months from the index nonunion procedure and 24 months from the initial injury. At a mean of 16 weeks (range 9–31 weeks), 84% (n = 41) were noted to be healed per computed tomography and there was significant improvement in scaphoid alignment and carpal height in terms of the revised carpal height ratio, scaphoid height-to-length ratio, scapholunate angle, and radiolunate angle, from preoperative to postoperative. For the 8 scaphoid nonunions that failed free medial femoral condyle VBG reconstruction, there was no significant association between failure and mean patient age, smoking status, body mass index, time from previous failed nonunion surgery, proximal pole fracture size, presence of fragmentation, cystic change, or degenerative change. However, a greater lateral intrascaphoid angle after free medial femoral condyle reconstruction was predictive of failure, with a mean of 23° in scaphoids that failed to heal compared with 14° in those that did ($P = .03$).[44]

Yet, there are limitations to the indications of a free medial femoral condyle VBG. Previous studies suggest using the free medial femoral condyle VBG only when the proximal pole of the scaphoid is large enough to accept an HCS or a K-wire or K-wires, has an intact cartilaginous shell, and is free from fragmentation.[12,53,54] If the characteristics of the proximal pole scaphoid is beyond these indications for a free medial femoral condyle VBG, then the free osteochondral medial femoral condyle trochlear VBG could be used. In these situations, a salvage procedure such as a proximal row carpectomy or scaphoidectomy and 4 corner arthrodesis may be the only other options for the patient. Elevation of the free medial femoral condyle VBG not only provides a rich blood supply via the transverse branch of the descending genicular artery and its branching periosteal vessels that supply the trochlea but also the graft allows for reconstruction of the proximal pole of the scaphoid by careful harvesting of the trochlear cartilage, which can effectively replicate the same radius of curvature as the scaphoid fossa.[12,55,56] Burger and colleagues[57] noted successful scaphoid reconstruction and restoration of carpal alignment with the free medial femoral trochlear VBG in 15 of 16 proximal pole scaphoid nonunions at a mean follow-up of 14 months.

PITFALLS OF THE LITERATURE

Composing a treatment algorithm based on the current body of literature for the management of scaphoid nonunions remains fraught with difficulty. Few definitions have been agreed on in the literature with respect to scaphoid nonunion avascularity, which makes comparisons difficult. For example, a multitude of options have been described for diagnosing AVN of the proximal scaphoid, including MRI, computed tomography, standard radiography, histopathologic assessment, and intraoperative vascularity, yet no single diagnostic method has been universally accepted. Furthermore, Rancy and colleagues[30] found no correlation between these diagnostic modalities, making the comparison of study results across the literature increasingly difficult. The definition of scaphoid union within the literature remains varied, thereby making comparison of study outcomes difficult as well. Moreover, the quality of scaphoid nonunion literature is poor, with retrospective case series and cohorts making up most of the evidence. Most of these studies contain heterogenous or unclear patient populations, scaphoid nonunion characteristics, and treatment groups, which can make it difficult to establish evidence-based treatment recommendations.

Treatment Recommendations for Scaphoid Nonunion Reconstruction

Given the decreased union rates in the setting of AVN or cases of previously failed nonvascularized bone grafting, the authors recommend the use of a

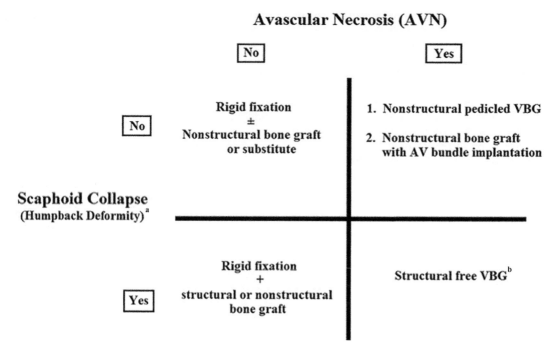

Fig. 2. Treatment recommendations for the use of nonvascularized bone grafts and VBGs in the management of scaphoid nonunions. [a] Lateral intrascaphoid angle greater than 45°. [b] Medial femoral condyle or trochlea-based free VBG based on the size and structure of the remaining proximal pole of the scaphoid with minimal to no degenerative changes. AV, arteriovenous.

VBG in these situations. Therefore, establishing the diagnosis of AVN in the treatment of scaphoid nonunion remains critical in guiding treatment. Advanced imaging, including computed tomography and MRI, may assist in the diagnosis; however, even when used, cases may still go undetected.[58,59] As such, the gold standard still remains visualizing the absence of punctate bleeding on tourniquet letdown at time of operative fixation.[29] **Fig. 2** illustrates the authors' recommended treatment algorithm for the management of scaphoid nonunions.

SUMMARY

Careful evaluation and diagnosis of scaphoid nonunions is critical in guiding treatment. Not every scaphoid nonunion requires a VBG; however, in the presence of AVN or previous bone nonvascularized bone graft failure, a VBG should be used to optimize revascularization and fracture-healing biology while correcting the humpback deformity. The authors recommend following basic tenants in the treatment of scaphoid nonunions, including removing the fibrous nonunion, excavation of sclerotic cancellous bone, insertion of autogenous bone graft, restoration of scaphoid length and carpal alignment, achieving rigid fixation, and (if

necessary) providing vascularity to the proximal pole in the setting of AVN. Through a combination of thorough evaluation and guided treatment, the outcomes of patients with scaphoid nonunion and proximal pole AVN can be improved with incorporation of a VBG.

REFERENCES

1. Moon ES, Dy CJ, Derman P, et al. Management of nonunion following surgical management of scaphoid fractures: current concepts. J Am Acad Orthop Surg 2013;21:548–57.
2. Dias JJ, Brenkel IJ, Finlay DB. Patterns of union in fractures of the waist of the scaphoid. J Bone Joint Surg Br 1989;71(2):307–10.
3. Gelberman RH, Menon J. The vascularity of the scaphoid bone. J Hand Surg Am 1980;5(5):508–13.
4. Kakar S, Bishop Shin AY. Role of vascularized bone grafts in the treatment of scaphoid nonunions associated with proximal pole avascular necrosis and carpal collapse. J Hand Surg Am 2011;36A:722–5.
5. Payatakes A, Sotereanos DG. Pedicled vascularized bone grafts for scaphoid and lunate reconstruction. J Am Acad Orthop Surg 2009;17:744–55.
6. Mack GR, Bosse MJ, Gelberman RH, et al. The natural history of scaphoid non-union. J Bone Joint Surg Am 1984;66(4):504–9.

7. Szabo RM, Manske D. Displaced fractures of the scaphoid. Clin Orthop Relat Res 1988;230:30–8.

8. Eddeland A, Eiken O, Hellgren E, et al. Fractures of the scaphoid. Scand J Plast Reconstr Surg 1975;9:234–9.

9. Cooney WP 3rd, Dobyns JH, Linscheid RL. Nonunion of the scaphoid: analysis of the results from bone grafting. J Hand Surg 1980;5:343–54.

10. Dias JJ. Definition of union after acute fracture and surgery for fracture nonunion of the scaphoid. J Hand Surg 2001;26B:321–5.

11. Osterman AL, Mikulics M. Scaphoid nonunion. Hand Clin 1988;4:437–55.

12. Rhee PC, Jones DB Jr, Shin AY, et al. Evaluation and treatment of scaphoid nonunions: a critical analysis review. JBJS Rev 2014;2(7):e4.

13. El-Karef EA. Corrective osteotomy for symptomatic scaphoid nonunion. Injury 2005;36(12):1440–8.

14. Ruby LK, Stinson J, Belsky MR. The natural history of scaphoid non0union. A review of fifty-five cases. J Bone Joint Surg Am 1985;67(3):428–32.

15. Pao VS, Chang J. Scaphoid nonunion: diagnosis and treatment. Plast Reconstr Surg 2003;112:1666–76.

16. Slade JF 3rd, Geissler WB, Gutow AP, et al. Percutaneous internal fixation of slected scaphoid nonunions with an arthroscopically assisted dorsal approach. J Bone Joint Surg Am 2003;85(Suppl 4):20–32.

17. Mahmoud M, Koptan W. Percutaneous screw fixation without bone grafting for established scaphoid nonunion with substantial bone loss. J Bone Joint Surg Br 2011;93(7):932–6.

18. Kim JK, Kim JO, Lee SY. Volar percutaneous screw fixation for scaphoid waist delayed union. Clin Orthop Relat Res 2010;468(4):1066–71.

19. Amadio PC, Berquist TH, Smith DK, et al. Scaphoid malunion. J Hand Surg Am 1989;14(4):679–87.

20. Merrell GA, Wolfe SW, Slade JF 3rd. Treatment of scaphoid nonunions: quantitative meta-analysis of the literature. J Hand Surg Am 2002;27A:685–91.

21. Tambe AD, Cutler L, Murali SR, et al. In scaphoid non-union, does the source of graft affect outcome? Iliac crest versus distal end of radius bone graft. J Hand Surg Br 2006;31(1):47–51.

22. Sayegh ET, Strauch RJ. Graft choice in the management of unstable scaphoid nonunion: a systematic review. J Hand Surg Am 2014;39(8):1500–6.

23. Russe O. Fracture of the carpal navicular; diagnosis, non-operative treatment and operative treatment. J Bone Joint Surg Am 1960;42:759–68.

24. Fernandez DL. Anterior bone grafting and conventional lag screw fixation to treat scaphoid nonunions. J Hand Surg Am 1990;15(1):140–7.

25. Yasuda M, Ando Y, Masada K. Treatment of scaphoid nonunion using volar biconcave cancellous bone grafting. Hand Surg 2007;12(2):135–40.

26. Daly K, Gill P, Magnussen PA, et al. Established nonunion of the scaphoid treated by volar wedge grafting and Herbert screw fixation. J Bone Joint Surg Br 1996;78(4):530–4.

27. Arora R, Lutz M, Zimmermann R, et al. Free vascularized bone graft for recalcitrant avascular nonunion of the scaphoid. J Bone Joint Surg Br 2010;92(2):224–9.

28. Robbins RR, Carter PR. Iliac crest bone grafting and Herbert screw fixation of nonunions of the scaphoid with avascular proximal poles. J Hand Surg 1995;20A:818–31.

29. Green DP. The effect of avascular necrosis on Russe bone grafting for scaphoid nonunion. J Hand Surg 1985;10A(5):597–605.

30. Rancy SK, Swanstrom MM, DiCarlo ED, et al. Success of scaphoid nonunion surgery is independent of proximal pole vascularity. J Hand Surg Br 2018;43(1):32–40.

31. Derby BM, Murray PM, Shin AY, et al. Vascularized bone grafts for the treatment of carpal bone pathology. Hand 2013;8:27–40.

32. Dell PC, Burchardt H, Glowczewskie FP Jr. A roentgenographic, biomechanical, and histological evaluation of vascularize and non-vascularized segmental fibular canine autografts. J Bone Joint Surg Am 1985;67(1):105–12.

33. Shaffer JW, Field GA, Goldberg VM, et al. Fate of vascularized and nonvascularized autografts. Clin Orthop Relat Res 1985;197:32–43.

34. Goldberg VM, Shaffer JW, Field G, et al. Biology of vascularized bone grafts. Orthop Clin North Am 1987;18(2):197–205.

35. Sunagawa T, Bishop AT, Muramatsu K. Role of conventional and vascularized bone grafts in scaphoid nonunion with avascular necrosis: a canine experimental study. J Hand Surg Am 2000;25:849–59.

36. Muramatsu K, Bishop A. Cell repopulation in vascularized bone grafts. J Orthop Res 2002;20:772–8.

37. Tu YK, Bishop AT, Kato T, et al. Experimental carpal reverse-flow pedicle vascularized bone grafts. Part II: bone blood flow measurement by radioactive labeled microspheres in a canine model. J Hand Surg Am 2000;25:46–54.

38. Nakamura R, Tsuge S, Watanabe K, et al. Radial wedge osteotomy for Kiebock disease. J Bone Joint Surg Am 1991;73(9):1391–6.

39. Al-Jabri T, Mannan A, Giannoudis P. The use of the free vascularized bone graft for nonunion of the scaphoid: a systematic review. J Orthop Surg Res 2014;9(21):1–9.

40. Pinder RM, Brkljac M, Rix L, et al. Treatment of scaphoid nonunion: a systematic review of the existing evidence. J Hand Surg Am 2015;40(9):1797–805.

41. Waitayawinyu T, McCallister W, Katolik L, et al. Outcome after vascularized bone grafting of

scaphoid nonunions with avascular necrosis. J Hand Surg Am 2009;34A:387–94.

42. Zaidemberg C, Siebert JW, Angrigiani C. A new vascularized bone graft for scaphoid nonunion. J Hand Surg Am 1991;16A:474–8.

43. Sheetz K, Bishop A, Berger R. The arterial blood supply of the distal radius and ulna and its potential use in vascularized pedicled bone grafts. J Hand Surg Am 1995;20:902–14.

44. Pulos N, Kollitz KM, Bishop AT, et al. Free vascularized medial femoral condyle bone graft after failed scaphoid nonunion surgery. J Bone Joint Surg Am 2018;100:1379–86.

45. Chang M, Bishop A, Moran SL, et al. The outcomes and complications of 1,2-intercompartmental supraretinacular artery pedicled vascularized bone grafting of scaphoid nonunions. J Hand Surg Am 2006; 31:387–96.

46. Malizos KN, Dailiana ZH, Kirou M, et al. Longstanding nonunions of scaphoid fractures with bone loss: successful reconstruction with vascularized bone grafts. J Hand Surg Br 2001;26(4):330–4.

47. Kollitz KM, Pulos N, Bishop AT, et al. Primary medial femoral condyle vascularized bone graft for scaphoid nonunions with carpal collapse and proximal pole avascular necrosis. J Hand Surg Eur Vol 2018. [Epub ahead of print].

48. Dailiana Z, Malizos K, Zachos V, et al. Vascularized bone grafts from the palmar radius for the treatment of waist nonunions of the scaphoid. J Hand Surg Am 2006;31:397–404.

49. Kawai H, Yamamoto K. Pronator quadratus pedicled bone graft for old scaphoid fractures. J Bone Joint Surg Br 1988;70B:829–31.

50. Mathoulin C, Haerle M. Vascularized bone graft from the palmar carpal artery for treatment of scaphoid nonunion. J Hand Surg Br 1998;23B:318–23.

51. Mathoulin CL, Haerle M. Technique: vascularized bone grafts from the volar distal radius to treat scaphoid nonunion. J Hand Surg Am 2004;4(1): 4–10.

52. Doi K, Oda T, Soo-Heong T, et al. Free vascularized bone graft for nonunion of the scaphoid. J Hand Surg Am 2000;25(3):507–19.

53. Jones DB Jr, Burger H, Bishop AT, et al. Treatment of scaphoid waist nonunions with an avascular proximal pole and carpal collapse. A comparison of two vascularized bone grafts. J Bone Joint Surg Am 2008;90(12):2616–25.

54. Larson AN, Bishop AT, Shin AY. Free medial femoral condyle bone grafting for scaphoid nonunions with humpback deformity and proximal pole avascular necrosis. Tech Hand Up Extrem Surg 2007;11(4): 246–58.

55. Iorio ML, Masden DL, Higgins JP. The limits of medial femoral condyle corticoperiosteal flaps. J Hand Surg Am 2011;36(10):1592–6.

56. Hugon S, Konickx A, Barbier O. Vascularized osteochondral graft from the medial femoral trochlea: anatomical study and clinical perspectives. Surg Radiol Anat 2010;32(9):817–25.

57. Burger HK, Windhofer C, Gaggl AJ, et al. Vascularized medial femoral trochlea osteocartilaginous flap reconstruction of proximal pole scaphoid nonunions. J Hand Surg Am 2013;38(4):201–5.

58. Schmitt R, Christopoulos G, Wagner M, et al. Avascular necrosis of the proximal fragment in scaphoid nonunion: is intravenous contrast agent necessary in MRI? Eur J Radiol 2011;77(2):222–7.

59. Willems WF, Alberton GM, Bishop AT, et al. Vascularized bone grafting in a canine carpal avascular necrosis model. Clin Orthop Relat Res 2011;469(10): 2831–7.

Does Anyone Need a Vascularized Graft?

Schneider K. Rancy, BA[a], Gernot Schmidle, MD[b], Scott W. Wolfe, MD[c],*

KEYWORDS

- Scaphoid nonunion • Vascularity • Avascular necrosis • Ischemia • Infarction
- Vascularized bone graft • Nonvascularized bone graft • Creeping substitution

KEY POINTS

- Many hand surgeons argue that vascularized bone grafting is indicated in proximal pole avascular necrosis, prior failed surgery, or long-standing nonunion.
- There is no evidence to show significant differences in union rate or time to union between vascularized and nonvascularized grafting.
- Current diagnostic tools do not accurately reflect proximal pole vascular status and may blur outcome comparisons between vascularized and nonvascularized bone grafting.
- Future studies should include histologic confirmation of proximal pole vascular status for purposes of stratification and valid outcome comparisons.
- Future comparative studies should control for proximal fragment size, fixation method, bony defects, and distal pole vascularity to better define absolute indications for vascularized bone grafting.

INTRODUCTION

The proximal pole is considered at risk for avascular necrosis (AVN) after fracture nonunion because of disruption of the scaphoid's intraosseous retrograde blood flow.[1–3] Proximal pole AVN reportedly occurs in 13% to 50% of scaphoid fractures, with a higher frequency in proximal fifth fractures.[4–6] Proximal pole vascularity has been identified as an important prognostic factor capable of predicting bony healing.[7–10]

Traditionally, nonvascularized bone grafts (NVBGs) with or without internal fixation have proved to be effective for scaphoid nonunion (SNU) treatment.[1,3,11–14] NVBG has undergone considerable technical evolution since Russe's[1] 1960 modification of Matti's technique. Vascularized bone grafts (VBGs) have recently gained popularity as an alternative surgical treatment.[15–17] Various VBG techniques have been described, including the 1,2 intercompartmental supraretinacular artery (1,2 ICSRA) graft,[18] the volar carpal artery (Mathoulin) graft,[19,20] the free tricortical iliac crest graft,[21] and the medial femoral condyle (MFC) graft.[22,23] Several investigators have advocated for obligatory VBG in proximal pole AVN, citing concerns of insufficient healing potential with traditional NVBG techniques.[18,24,25] However, clinical parameters for diagnosis of AVN are variable and not widely accepted.[17,26] Other investigators have suggested prior failed surgery, proximal pole location, fracture instability, and structural defects (humpback deformity, dorsal intercalated segmental instability [DISI], or fragmentation) as indications for VBG,[23,27–29] but there is little consensus around treatment algorithms. Consequently, there is considerable controversy regarding whether and when VBG should be used for SNU treatment.[2,3,17,26,30,31]

Disclosures: None.
[a] College of Medicine, SUNY Downstate Medical Center, 1160 Ocean Avenue, Apt 5F, Brooklyn, NY 11230, USA;
[b] Department of Trauma Surgery, Medical University Innsbruck, Anichstraße 35, Innsbruck 6020, Austria;
[c] Hand and Upper Extremity Service, Hospital for Special Surgery, Weill Medical College of Cornell University, 535 East 70th Street, New York, NY 10021, USA
* Corresponding author.
E-mail address: wolfes@hss.edu

Hand Clin 35 (2019) 323–344
https://doi.org/10.1016/j.hcl.2019.03.005

This article addresses the available evidence and examines the role of VBG in SNU treatment. It identifies important factors that influence healing, derives conclusions from an analysis of the literature, and proposes areas for further research.

LITERATURE REVIEW
Vascularity

Proximal pole AVN is generally deemed by most investigators to be the main indication for vascularized bone grafting. In clinical practice, the term AVN is used for a wide spectrum of conditions of assumed circulatory compromise.[2,9] Büchler and Nagy[2] defined AVN as histologically proven "death of bone substance from anoxia and its sequelae" and proposed a classification scheme based on histology. In class 1 AVN, the proximal fragment is temporarily deprived of intraosseous circulation and central marrow necrosis occurs while trabecular structure is preserved as scaffolding for new osteoid formation. In class 2, if circulatory disruption or mechanical loading continues, trabecular collapse and fragmentation (infarction) occur. The surrounding well-vascularized tissues promote focal bone resorption and fibrosis. In class 2A, central fragmentation, fibrosis of trabecular remnants, and cystic lesions are present with poor osteogenic activity. In class 2B, compression and resorption cease. Necrotic bone may then revascularize and undergo replacement with viable bone, but structural integrity cannot be regained.

Several diagnostic approaches are applied to assess vascularity. Characteristic features on plain radiographs can suggest AVN, including sclerosis, fragmentation, or collapse, but cannot accurately predict vascularity.[25,32] In 1985, Green[7] famously defined AVN as absent punctate bleeding on intraoperative inspection. However, he noted many instances in which histologic presence or absence of viable osteocytes did not agree with bleeding assessment. Nonetheless, many investigators have since defined AVN as absent bleeding when reporting SNU treatment outcomes, irrespective of bone grafting technique and type (Tables 1–5). Several investigators have also used absent bleeding as the reference standard for AVN when evaluating the diagnostic accuracy of other vascular assessment modalities, despite this parameter's shortcomings.

Günal and colleagues[9] compared T_1-weighted and T_2-weighted magnetic resonance (MR) signal intensity with punctate bleeding and found that the two parameters agreed in only 19 out of 32 SNUs. Fox and colleagues[33] likewise compared unenhanced T_1-weighted MR signal intensity with punctate bleeding in 29 SNUs and reported 55%

sensitivity, 94% specificity, and 79% accuracy. Donati and colleagues[34] reported similar numbers and further concluded that unenhanced MR was diagnostically superior to gadolinium-enhanced MR in 28 patients. There was no correlation between contrast enhancement and proximal pole trabecular composition on histology in their study (P>.05). In contrast, Schmitt and colleagues[35] compared unenhanced T_1-weighted and T_2-weighted MR signal intensity with contrast uptake against punctate bleeding in 88 SNUs. They concluded that contrast MRI had significantly improved sensitivity (76.5% vs 6.3%) and accuracy (94.3% vs 82.9%) compared with unenhanced MRI for proximal pole AVN (P<.001).

Bervian and colleagues[36] compared radiographic and computed tomography (CT) radiodensity, unenhanced T_1-weighted MR signal intensity, and punctate bleeding with histologic trabecular necrosis as the reference in 19 SNUs. The investigators qualitatively graded biopsy specimens based on the relative presence of osteoblasts, remodeling, necrotic myeloid tissue, and changes in trabecular surface but were unable to quantify necrosis. They found significant positive correlations between histology and radiographic findings, MRI, and punctate bleeding (P<.05), but qualitative assessment of CT radiodensity relative to the capitate on 1-mm to 3-mm slices did not correlate with histology.

Megerle and colleagues[10] reported a strong positive association between MR findings and punctate bleeding in 49 SNUs (P<.001). However, they found no significant correlation between contrast MRI assessment of proximal pole vascularity and their 90% union rate with NVBG and screw fixation in 60 patients (P = .47). Several other studies have also failed to show any correlation between union rate and vascularity as assessed with punctate bleeding and both unenhanced and contrast MRI.[9,37,38]

These findings show there is conflicting evidence about the ability of radiographs, CT, or MRI to accurately diagnose AVN preoperatively. Furthermore, although several diagnostic modalities exist for vascular assessment, the use of punctate bleeding as the reference standard makes their accuracy, sensitivity, and specificity indeterminate. The current ability to predict scaphoid vascularity is poor, and this may limit analyses of its effect on healing potential. The utility of VBG to compensate for poor vascularity is therefore uncertain.

Scaphoid Nonunion Treatment Outcomes

The authors reviewed the English-language literature on outcomes for both NVBG and VBG

Table 1
Nonvascularized bone graft case series outcomes

Investigators, Year	Vascular Assessment	PP Vascular Status	Proximal Fragment Size	PPª	Fixation	Union Assessment	Union Rate	Time to Union
Russe Type								
Green[7] 1985	BB, histology	AVN: 5 Fair/poor: 14 Good: 26 (by BB)	Proximal third, proximal half, proximal two-thirds	9 out of 45 (20%)	None	Radiographs	34 out of 45 (75%)	5.33 mo
Stark et al,[39] 1987	Radiographs	Sclerosis, bone cysts: 27	Proximal third, proximal half, proximal two-thirds	3 out of 27 (11%)	None	Radiographs	22 out of 27 (81%)	NR (follow-up 12 y)
Warren-Smith & Barton,[40] 1988; Barton,[41] 1997	NR	NR	NR	4 out of 28 (14%)	K-wires in 5, none in 23	Radiographs	Certain: 15 out of 28 (60%) Uncertain: 1 out of 28 (4%)	NR (follow-up 3.6 y)
Barton,[41] 1997	BB	AVN: 3	NR	4 out of 28 (14%)	None	Radiographs	Certain: 15 out of 28 (60%) Uncertain: 7 out of 28 (25%)	NR (follow-up 2.2 y)
Total	—	AVN: 8 out of 100 (8%)	—	20 out of 128 (16%)	—	—	86 out of 128 (67%)	—
Cavitation and Cancellous Graft with Fixation								
Stark et al,[11] 1988	Radiographs	AVN: 25	Proximal third, proximal half, proximal two-thirds	32 out of 151 (21%)	K-wires	CT, radiographs, tomographs	147 out of 151 (97%) AVN subgroup: 21 out of 24 (88%)	17 wk

(continued on next page)

Table 1
(continued)

Investigators, Year	Vascular Assessment	PP Vascular Status	Proximal Fragment Size	PP[a]	Fixation	Union Assessment	Union Rate	Time to Union
Warren-Smith & Barton,[40] 1988; Barton,[41] 1997	NR	NR	NR	1 out of 32 (3%)	Herbert screw	Radiographs	Certain: 25 out of 32 (78%) Uncertain: 1 out of 32 (3%)	NR (follow-up 4.2 y)
Trumble,[42] 1990	BB, histology, MRI w/o contrast, radiographs, tetracycline fluorescence	AVN: 4 (by histology)	Proximal half	0 out of 9 (0%)	Herbert screw (8) or K-wire (1)	Trispiral tomographs	7 out of 9 (78%) Screw: 6 out of 8 (75%) K-wire: 1 out of 1 (100%)	NR (follow-up 15 mo)
Robbins,[8] 1995	BB	AVN: 5	Proximal third	5 out of 5 (100%)	Herbert screw	Radiographs	Bony: 2 out of 5 (40%) Incomplete/fibrous: 3 out of 5 (60%)	NR (follow-up 31 mo)
Barton,[41] 1997	NR	NR	NR	NR	K-wires	Radiographs	Certain: 15 out of 27 (56%) Uncertain: 6 out of 27 (22%)	NR (follow-up 2.4 y)
Barton,[41] 1997	NR	NR	NR	15 out of 15 (100%)	Herbert screw	Radiographs	Certain: 6 out of 15 (40%) Uncertain: 4 out of 15 (27%)	NR (follow-up 2 y)

Study		AVN	Location		Fixation	Imaging	Union	Follow-up
Morgan et al,[43] 1997	Histology, MRI w/o contrast, radiographs	AVN: 0 Viable: 6 (by histology and MRI)	Proximal third, proximal half	3 out of 6 (50%)	Herbert screw	CT	6 out of 6 (100%)	4.3 mo
Schmitt et al,[35] 2011	BB, MRI with and w/o contrast	AVN: 17 Compromised: 29 Normal: 42 (by BB)	NR	NR	Herbert or mini-Herbert screw	CT (in 34), radiographs (in all)	76 out of 88 (86%)	9–16 mo
Cohen et al,[44] 2013	CT, radiographs	All viable	Proximal half	0 out of 12 (0%)	Screw	CT	12 out of 12 (100%)	NR
Putnam et al,[45] 2018	BB	AVN: 13	Proximal third, proximal half	12 out of 13 (92%)	Locking plate	CT	13 out of 13 (100%)	20 wk (range, 12–30 wk)
Kim et al,[6] 2018	CT, BB, MRI w/o contrast, radiographs	AVN: 13 (by BB and MRI)	Proximal third, proximal half	10 out of 13 (77%)	K-wires	CT and radiographs	12 out of 13 (92%)	NR
Rancy et al,[38] 2018	BB, histology, MRI w/o contrast	AVN (>50% necrosis): 6 Impaired (10%–50% necrosis): 8 Normal (<10% necrosis): 1 (by histology)	Proximal fifth (1), proximal third, proximal half, proximal two-thirds	8 out of 16 (50%)	Herbert screw	CT	15 out of 16 (94%)	12 wk (range, 7–16 wk)
Total	—	AVN: 82 out of 311 (26%)	—	86 out of 272 (32%)	—	—	336 out of 387 (87%)	—
Distal Radius or Iliac Crest Structural Corticocancellous Graft with Fixation								
Trumble,[42] 1990	BB, histology, MRI w/o contrast, radiographs, tetracycline fluorescence	AVN: 2 (by histology)	Proximal half	0 out of 3 (0%)	Herbert screw (2) or K-wire (1)	Trispiral tomographs	2 out of 3 (67%) Screw: 2 out of 2 (100%) K-wires: 0 out of 1 (0%)	NR (follow-up 15 mo)

(continued on next page)

Table 1
(continued)

Investigators, Year	Vascular Assessment	PP Vascular Status	Proximal Fragment Size	PP[a]	Fixation	Union Assessment	Union Rate	Time to Union
Nakamura et al,[46] 1993	Radiographs	Sclerosis, cystic changes: 11 (5 with PP collapse)	Proximal third, proximal half, proximal two-thirds	7 out of 50 (14%)	Herbert screw	Radiographs and motion study	47 out of 50 (94%)	NR (follow-up 20 mo, range 12–72 mo)
Robbins,[8] 1995	BB	AVN: 12	Proximal half, proximal two-thirds	0 out of 12 (0%)	Herbert screw	Radiographs	Bony: 7 out of 12 (58%) Incomplete/fibrous: 4 out of 12 (33%)	NR (follow-up 31 mo)
Morgan et al,[43] 1997	Histology, MRI w/o contrast, radiographs	AVN: 4 Viable: 9 (by histology and MRI)	Proximal third, proximal half	1 out of 13 (8%) (21%)	Herbert screw	CT	11 out of 13 (85%)	5.6 mo
Ritter & Giachino,[47] 2000	Radiographs	AVN: 3 Sclerosis, cystic changes: 21	Proximal fifth (1), proximal third, proximal half, proximal two-thirds	5 out of 34 (14%)	Herbert screw (5), AO screw (5), or K-wires (24)	Radiographs	23 out of 34 (68%) Herbert: 2 out of 5 (40%) AO: 4 out of 5 (80%) K-wires: 16 out of 24 (67%)	8.2 mo
Matsuki et al,[48] 2011	MRI w/o contrast, radiographs	Preserved: 9 Poor: 2 (by MRI and/or radiographs)	Proximal third	11 out of 11 (100%)	Herbert, mini-Herbert, or Herbert-type screw	Radiographs	11 out of 11 (100%)	12–24 wk
Megerle et al,[10] 2011	BB, MRI with contrast	AVN: 7 Compromised: 19 Normal: 23 (by BB)	Proximal third, proximal half, proximal two-thirds	25 out of 60 (42%)	Herbert screw	Radiographs, CT if needed	54 out of 60 (90%)	12 wk

Kim et al,[6] 2018	CT, BB, MRI w/o contrast, radiographs	AVN: 11 (by BB and MRI)	Proximal half	0 out of 11 (0%)	Herbert screw (8) or K-wires (3)	CT and radiographs	10 out of 11 (91%) Herbert: 8 out of 8 (100%) K-wires: 2 out of 3 (67%)	NR
Rancy et al,[38] 2018	BB, histology, MRI w/o contrast	AVN (>50% necrosis): 8 Impaired (10%–50% necrosis): 8 Normal (<10% necrosis): 1 (by histology)	Proximal third, proximal half, proximal two-thirds	1 out of 19 (5%)	Herbert screw	CT	19 out of 19 (100%)	13 wk (range, 6–38)
Total	—	AVN: 49 out of 211 (23%)	—	50 out of 213 (23%)	—	—	184 out of 213 (86%)	—
Graft Type NR								
Sakuma et al,[49] 1995	MRI w/o contrast, radiographs	Normal/impaired: 30 Ischemic: 2 (by MRI)	Proximal third, proximal half, proximal two-thirds	4 out of 32 (13%)	Herbert screw	Radiographs	29 out of 32 (91%)	NR (follow-up 14 mo)
Günal et al,[9] 1999	BB, MRI w/o contrast	AVN: 7 Normal: 11 (by BB)	NR	NR	Herbert screw or K-wires	NR	17 out of 18 (94%)	NR
Total	—	AVN: 7 out of 50 (14%)	—	4 out of 32 (13%)	—	—	46 out of 50 (92%)	—

Abbreviations: BB, bleeding bone; K-wire, Kirschner wire; NR, not reported; PP, proximal pole; w/o, without.
a Proximal third or smaller.

Table 2
Vascularized bone grafts case series outcomes

Investigators, Year	Vascular Assessment	PP Vascular Status	Proximal Fragment Size	PP[a]	Fixation	Union Assessment	Union Rate	Time to Union
1,2 ICSRA								
Zaidemberg et al,[18] 1991	NR	NR	NR	NR	K-wires	Radiographs	11 out of 11 (100%)	6.2 wk (range, 5–8 wk)
Boyer et al,[52] 1998	CT, radiographs	AVN: 10 (by CT and radiographs)	Proximal third	10 out of 10 (100%)	Herbert screw and K-wires	CT	6 out of 10 (60%)	4.6 mo
Steinmann et al,[53] 2002	BB	AVN: 4	Proximal third, proximal half	8 out of 14 (57%)	Herbert screw (3), K-wires (10), or none (1)	Radiographs and trispiral tomography	14 out of 14 (100%)	11.1 wk (range, 8–16 wk)
Straw et al,[54] 2002	BB	AVN: 16 Poor: 2 Normal: 4	Proximal third, proximal half	17 out of 22 (77%)	Mini-Herbert screw (7) or K-wires (15)	CT (5), radiographs (17)	6 out of 22 (27%) Screws: 1 out of 7 (14%) K-wire: 5 out of 15 (33%)	8–16 wk
Chang et al,[27] 2006	BB, MRI unspecified, radiographs	AVN: 24 No AVN: 23 (by BB)	Proximal third, proximal half	25 out of 48 (52%)	Cannulated screw (26), K-wires (15), or both (4)	CT or tomographs	34 out of 48 (71%) Screws: 23 out of 26 (88%) K-wires: 8 out of 15 (53%)	15.6 wk

Henry,[55] 2007	BB, MRI w/o contrast	AVN: 15 (by BB and MRI)	NR	NR	Compression screw and K-wires	CT	No AVN subgroup: 21 out of 23 (91%) Screws: 17 out of 17 K-wires: 4 out of 6 (67%)	14 wk (range, 8–40 wk)
							AVN subgroup: 12 out of 24 (50%) Screws: 5 out of 8 (63%) K-wires: 4 out of 9 (44%)	18 wk (range, 8–30 wk)
							15 out of 15 (100%)	11.5 wk
Jones et al,[23] 2008	BB, CT, MRI with contrast	AVN: 10 (by BB)	Proximal half	0 out of 10 (0%)	K-wires (7) or screw and K-wires (3)	CT, radiographs, trispiral tomograms	4 out of 10 (40%) K-wires: 3 out of 7 (43%) K-wires + screw: 1 out of 3 (33%)	19 wk
Waitayawinyu et al,[56] 2009	BB, MRI w/o contrast	AVN: 30 (by BB and MRI)	Proximal third, proximal half	11 out of 30 (37%)	Herbert-Whipple or Acutrak cannulated screw	CT	28 out of 30 (93%)	5.1 mo
Lim et al,[57] 2013	BB	AVN: 21 (by BB)	Proximal third or smaller	21 out of 21 (100%)	K-wires	Radiographs, CT (in 8 cases)	18 out of 21 (86%)	14 wk (range, 8–28 wk)

(continued on next page)

Table 2
(*continued*)

Investigators, Year	Vascular Assessment	PP Vascular Status	Proximal Fragment Size	PP[a]	Fixation	Union Assessment	Union Rate	Time to Union
Morris et al,[58] 2018	BB, CT, MRI unspecified, radiographs	AVN: 7 Viable: 4 (by BB)	Proximal third or smaller	11 out of 11 (100%)	Headless compression screw	CT	11 out of 11 (100%)	11.44 wk (range, 8–13.86 wk)
Total	—	AVN: 137 out of 181 (76%)	—	103 out of 163 (63%)	—	—	147 out of 192 (77%)	—
Volar Carpal Artery Pedicle (Mathoulin)								
Kuhlmann et al,[19] 1987	NR	NR	NR	NR	K-wires	Radiographs, tomograms	3 out of 3 (100%)	2 mo
Mathoulin & Haerle,[20] 1998	NR	NR	Proximal half	0 out of 17 (0%)	Screw	Radiographs	17 out of 17 (100%)	60 d
Dailiana et al,[59] 2006	CT, MRI with and w/o contrast	AVN: 1 (by MRI)	Proximal half	0 out of 9 (0%)	K-wires	MRI with and w/o contrast	9 out of 9 (100%)	6–8 wk
Gras & Mathoulin,[60] 2011	NR	NR	Proximal third, proximal half	24 out of 111 (22%)	Screw	Radiographs	104 out of 111 (94%)	10 wk
—	—	NA	—	24 out of 137 (8%)	—	—	133 out of 140 (95%)	—
Free Iliac Crest								
Harpf et al,[62] 2001	BB	AVN: 26	Small pole	26 out of 60	K-wire	Radiographs	55 out of 60 (92%) AVN: 24 out of 26 (92%) 4-y+ SNU: 19 out of 21 (90%) Failed surgery: 12 out of 13 (92%)	NR (follow-up 7.4 y)

Study	Diagnosis Method	AVN	Location	AVN Healed	Fixation	Imaging	Union	Time to Union
Gabl et al,[61] 1999	BB, histology, radiographs	AVN: 15 (by BB, histology, and radiographs)	Proximal third	15 out of 15 (100%)	Temporary pin	Radiographs	12 out of 15 (80%)	NR (follow-up 16 mo)
Arora et al,[63] 2010	BB, MRI with contrast	AVN: 21 (by BB and MRI)	Proximal third, proximal half	6 out of 21 (29%)	K-wire	Radiographs	16 out of 21 (76%)	17 wk (waist), 21 wk (proximal pole)
Total	—	AVN: 62 out of 96 (65%)	—	47 out of 96 (49%)	—	—	83 out of 96 (86%)	—
Medial Femoral Condyle								
Doi et al,[22] 2000	BB, MRI w/o contrast	AVN: 10 (by BB)	Proximal third, proximal half	4 out of 10 (40%)	K-wires	Radiographs and tomograms	10 out of 10 (100%)	12 wk
Jones et al,[23] 2008	BB, CT, MRI with contrast	AVN: 12 (by BB)	Proximal half	0 out of 12 (0%)	Cannulated screw (7), K-wires (4), or both (1)	CT, radiographs, trispiral tomograms	12 out of 12 (100%)	13 wk
Pulos et al,[29] 2018	BB	AVN: 49 (by BB)	NR	NR	Screw (21), K-wires (22), or both (6)	CT	41 out of 49 (84%)	16 wk (range, 9–31)
Total	—	AVN: 71 out of 71 (100%)	—	4 out of 22 (18%)	—	—	63 out of 71 (89%)	—

Abbreviation: NA, not available.
[a] Proximal third or smaller.

Table 3
Vascularized bone grafts versus nonvascularized bone grafts (all techniques): retrospective series

Author, Year	Sample Size (SNUs)	Vascular Assessment	PP Vascular Status	Proximal Fragment Size	% PP	Graft Type (VBG vs NVBG)	Fixation (VBG vs NVBG)	Union Assessment	Union Rate: VBG vs NVBG	Time to Union: VBG vs NVBG	Significance of Difference (Union Rate/ Time)
Hirche et al,[64] 2017	73	NR	VBG: 28 out of 28 avascular PP or PPN NVBG: 45 out of 45 unimpaired vascularity	NR	NR	1,2 ICSRA vs cortico-cancellous IC	Screw or K-wires vs screw or K-wires	Radiographs, or CT if unclear	21 out of 28 (75%) vs 37 out of 45 (82%)	NR	P = .555/NR

Abbreviations: IC, iliac crest; NR, not reported; PPN, proximal pole nonunion.

Table 4
Vascularized bone graft versus nonvascularized bone graft: systematic reviews

Investigators, Year	Sample Size (SNUs/Articles)	Vascular Assessment	PP Vascular Status	Proximal Fragment Size	% PP[a]	Graft Type (VBG vs NVBG)	Fixation (VBG vs NVBG)	Union Assessment	Union Rate: VBG vs NVBG	Time to Union: VBG vs NVBG	Difference Significance (Union Rate/Time)
Merrell et al,[30] 2002	64 out of 36	BB	AVN in all patients (by BB)	Proximal third, proximal half, proximal two-thirds	NR	Unspecified vs wedge	Screw or K-wires vs Screw	CT or tomographs in some, otherwise NR	30 out of 34 (88%) vs 14 out of 30 (47%)	NR	P<.0005/NR
Munk & Larsen,[65] 2004	5249 out of 147	NR	VBG: "almost exclusively" PP AVN or prior surgery NVBG: NR	Fracture line "in all parts" of scaphoid, highly variable	NR	DR, IC, MC vs DR, IC	VBG with and w/o screws, K-wires vs NVBG with screws, K-wires, pins, plates, staples	NR	301 out of 331 (91%) vs 2242 out of 2669 (84%)	10 vs 7 wk	NR/NR
Pinder et al,[17] 2015	1602 out of 48	Variable, unspecified	VBG: 68% NVBG: 40%	NR	NR	DR, IC, MC, MFC vs IC, DR, rib	Screw or K-wires vs screw, K-wires, or none	Variable, including radiographs alone, radiographs with CT, and/or MRI	479 out of 521 (92%) vs 874 out of 993 (88%)	13.8 vs 13.6 wk	NS/NR

(continued on next page)

Table 4
(continued)

Investiga-tors, Year	Sample Size (SNUs/ Articles	Vascular Assessment	PP Vascular Status	Proximal Fragment Size	% PP[a]	Graft Type (VBG vs NVBG)	Fixation (VBG vs NVBG)	Union Assessment	Union Rate: VBG vs NVBG	Time to Union: VBG vs NVBG	Difference Significance (Union Rate/ Time)
Ferguson et al,[26] 2016	5464 out of 144	BB, CT, MRI with and w/o contrast, radiographs	VBG: AVN in 292 NVBG: AVN in 236 (by variable modalities)	Proximal fifth, proximal third, proximal half, proximal two-thirds	NR	DR, IC, MC, MFC vs IC, DR	Screws, K-wires, none, or unspecified other vs screws, K-wires, none, or unspecified other	Variable, including radiographs, CT, or clinical examination	758 out of 902 (84%) vs 2662 out of 3327 (80%) AVN subgroup: 217 out of 292 (74%) vs 146 out of 236 (62%)	NR/NR; for pooled data, 45 mo (range, 1–456 mo)	NR/NR

Abbreviations: DR, distal radius; IC, iliac crest; MC, metacarpal; MFC, medial femoral condyle; NR, not reported; NS, not significant.
[a] Proximal third or smaller.

Table 5
Vascularized bone graft versus nonvascularized bone graft: prospective randomized studies

Investigators, Year	Sample Size (SNUs)	Vascular Assessment	PP Vascular Status	Proximal Fragment Size	% PP (VBG vs NVBG)	Graft Type (VBG vs NVBG)	Fixation (VBG vs NVBG)	Union Assessment	Union Rate: VBG vs NVBG	Time to Union: VBG vs NVBG	Significance of Difference (Union Rate/Time)
Braga-Silva et al,[31] 2008	80	BB (in 5 VBG patients), radiographs	VBG: 13 out of 35 (37%) sclerotic NVBG: 8 out of 45 (18%) sclerotic (by radiographs)	Proximal third, proximal half	12 out of 35 (34%) vs 12 out of 45 (27%)	1,2 ICSRA vs cortico-cancellous IC wedge	Herbert screws or K-wires vs Herbert screws	Radiographs	32 out of 35 (91%) vs 45 out of 45 (100%)	8 vs 8.9 wk	NR/$P = .135$
Ribak et al,[24] 2010	86	BB	VBG: 30 out of 46 (65%) with absent bleeding NVBG: 20 out of 40 (50%) with absent bleeding	Proximal third, proximal half, proximal two-thirds	21 out of 46 (46%) vs 16 out of 40 (40%)	1,2 ICSRA vs cortico-cancellous DR	K-wires vs K-wires	Radiographs	41 out of 46 (89.1%) vs 29 out of 40 (72.5%) PP subgroup: 19 out of 21 (90.5%) vs 11 out of 16 (68.8%)	9.7 vs 12.0 wk	$P = .024$/$P < .0001$ PP subgroup: $P = .09$/NR

Abbreviations: DR, distal radius; IC, iliac crest.

techniques. For each identified study, proximal pole vascular assessment and status, proximal fragment size, percentage proximal pole fractures per cohort, fixation type, union assessment modality (eg, radiographs, CT), union rate, and time to union were recorded. For studies using multiple techniques per series (eg, cancellous or cortico-cancellous NVBG), articles were stratified to separately report outcomes by graft type.

Nonvascularized bone graft case series
Table 1 shows outcomes for several different NVBG techniques. For Russe type[1] NVBG, AVN was present in 8% (8 out of 100) of SNUs and confirmed by absent punctate bleeding. Sixteen percent (20 out of 128) of SNUs were located in the proximal pole or more proximally. With no fixation in most cases, union was achieved in 67% (86 out of 128) as assessed by radiographs. However, it is generally agreed that rigid fixation is favored in modern SNU treatment, and these cases are presented for historical interest.

For cavitation and cancellous NVBG with internal fixation, AVN was present in 26% (82 out of 311) of SNUs according to absent punctate bleeding, MRI signal intensity and/or contrast uptake, and/or radiography. AVN was diagnosed with histologic section in only 3 studies (40 patients).[38,42,43] Proximal third or smaller fracture nonunions were seen in 32% (86 out of 272). According to radiography, tomography, and CT, union was achieved in 87% (336 out of 387) with screw or Kirschner wire (K-wire) fixation in most cases.

Similarly, outcomes were assessed for distal radius strut graft or iliac crest corticocancellous wedge NVBG with internal fixation, as first detailed by Fisk[50] and later modified by Fernandez.[12,51] AVN was present in 23% (49 out of 211) according to absent punctate bleeding, MRI signal intensity and/or contrast uptake, and/or radiography. Histologic sectioning was again only used in 3 studies. Proximal third or smaller nonunions were seen in 23% (50 out of 21). According to radiography, tomography, and CT, union was achieved in 86% (184 out of 213) with screw or K-wire fixation.

Two series[9,49] did not clearly describe the NVBG technique used. Union was achieved in 92% (46 out of 50) when AVN was present in 14% (7 out of 50) according to absent punctate bleeding and/or MRI. Overall, AVN was seen in 22% (146 out of 672) of SNUs but was verified with histologic section in only 3 studies,[38,42,43] accounting for 40 patients. When excluding historical reports without fixation, union occurred in 87% (566 out of 650). On subgroup analysis including patients with vascularity assessed by any modality, treated

with screw fixation,[6,38,43,44] and with union confirmed by CT, union was 96% (71 out of 74). Of these, 21 of 22 SNUs with AVN healed (95%).[6,38]

Vascularized bone graft case series
Table 2 shows outcomes for VBG according to several series. With the 1,2 ICSRA graft originally described by Zaidemberg,[18] AVN was present in 76% (137 out of 181) according to absent bleeding, MRI, radiography, and/or CT. When reported, proximal fragments comprised the proximal third or smaller in 63% (103 out of 163). Both screw and K-wire internal fixation were used and union was assessed with radiography, tomography, and/or CT. Union was achieved in 77% (147 out of 192).

For the volar carpal artery pedicled graft first reported by Kuhlman and colleagues,[19] AVN assessment was not routinely reported. Proximal third or smaller nonunions were seen in 8% (24 out of 137). With screw and K-wire fixation, union was achieved in 95% (133 out of 140).

When a free iliac crest VBG was used as first described by Pechlaner and colleagues,[21] AVN was present in 65% (62 out of 96) according to absent bleeding, MRI, and/or radiography, with histology being used in 1 study.[61] Proximal third or small nonunions comprised 49% (47 out of 96) of SNUs. With temporary pin or K-wire fixation, union was achieved in 86% (83 out of 96) according to radiography.

An MFC VBG was used in 71 SNUs. AVN was present in all cases (71 out of 71) according to absent punctate bleeding. When reported, proximal third or smaller nonunions occurred in 18% (4 out of 22). With screw and/or K-wire fixation, union was achieved in 89% (63 out of 71) according to radiography, tomography, and CT.

In general, AVN was present in 78% (270 out of 348), likely reflecting a preference for VBG in cases in which AVN is suspected, although histologic verification was used in only 1 series.[61] Union was seen in 85% (426 out of 499) overall with either screw or K-wire fixation. On subgroup analysis including patients with vascularity assessed by any modality, treated with screw fixation,[27,56,58] and union confirmed by CT, union was 93% (62 out of 67), equivalent to NVBG union rates in the same population. Of these, 40 of 45 SNUs with AVN healed (89%).[27,56,58]

Nonvascularized bone graft versus vascularized bone grafts (all techniques): retrospective series
A single retrospective cohort study[64] directly comparing NVBG versus VBG outcomes was

found and is shown in **Table 3**. The investigators compared 45 SNUs treated with a corticocancellous iliac crest NVBG with 28 SNUs treated with 1,2 ICSRA VBG. Grafts in both groups were stabilized with either a screw or K-wire construct. The investigators noted that NVBG was only used in cases of unimpaired vascularity, whereas VBG was exclusively for proximal AVN or proximal nonunion, but did not detail their vascular assessment modality. Union was reported in 82% of the NVBG group and 75% in the VBG group, a difference that did not reach statistical significance ($P = .5557$). The uncertain assessment of AVN in this study renders these results inconclusive.

Nonvascularized bone graft versus vascularized bone graft: systematic reviews

Several systematic reviews and meta-analyses compare the outcomes between NVBG and VBG. A summary of these findings is shown in **Table 4**.

Merrell and colleagues[30] reported a statistically significant difference in union rate ($P<.0005$) between NVBG (47%; 14 out of 30) and VBG (88%; 30 out of 34) when AVN was present in all patients according to absent punctate bleeding. However, these numbers are arguably small and the use of punctate bleeding for AVN assessment questions the validity of the conclusion. Munk and Larson[65] later reported 84% (2242 out of 2669) union for NVBG by 7 weeks compared with 91% (301 out of 331) union for VBG by 10 weeks, but VBG was used "almost exclusively" for proximal pole AVN or prior surgery, whereas vascularity in the NVBG was not explicitly detailed. Vascular assessment modality and statistical significance were not reported.

Pinder and colleagues[17] reviewed 1602 SNUs in 48 articles and reported AVN in 40% of NVBG patients compared with 68% in the VBG group according to various unspecified diagnostic modalities. Union was seen in 88% (874 out of 993) of the NVBG group by 13.6 weeks compared with 92% (479 out of 521) in the VBG group by 13.8 weeks, a non–statistically significant difference. In an even larger systematic review by Ferguson and colleagues,[26] the union rate for NVBG was 80% (2662 out of 3327) compared with 84% (758 out of 902) for VBG. On subgroup analysis of patients with purported AVN, union was 62% (146 out of 236) in NVBG patients compared with 74% (217 out of 292) in VBG patients. AVN was diagnosed with punctate bleeding, MRI, or CT across studies. Statistics comparing union rate were not reported. No systematic review detailed statistical comparisons for time to union.

These studies support the pooled data analyzed from case series in **Tables 1** and **2** and nonstatistically indicate equivalent union rates between NVBG and VBG. These studies also suggest higher union rates for VBG in a subgroup of patients with AVN. However, the multiplicity of diagnostic modalities calls into question the accuracy of AVN diagnosis and raises concerns about possible confounders such as instrumentation, proximal fragment size, structural defects (eg, humpback deformity), and union assessment modality.

Nonvascularized bone graft versus vascularized bone graft: evidence of randomized trials

Table 5 details variables and outcomes for 2 prospective randomized trials directly comparing NVBG and VBG in the setting of AVN.

Braga-Silva and colleagues[31] compared 45 patients undergoing structural corticocancellous iliac crest NVBG with Herbert screw fixation with 35 patients undergoing 1,2 ICSRA VBG with Herbert screw or K-wire fixation. AVN was predominantly diagnosed with radiographic sclerosis and was present in 18% of NVBG patients compared with 37% in VBG patients. Union was reported as 100% for NVBG by 8.9 weeks and 91% for VBG by 8 weeks. There was no significant difference in time to union ($P = .135$), but statistics for union rate were not reported.

In contrast, Ribak and colleagues[24] prospectively randomized 40 SNUs to corticocancellous distal radius NVBG with K-wires and 46 SNUs to 1,2 ICSRA VBG with K-wires. AVN was present in 50% of NVBG patients and 65% of VBG patients but was diagnosed by absent bleeding. Union for NVBG was 72.5% by 12 weeks and 89.1% by 9.7 weeks in the VBG group, a significant difference in union rate ($P = .024$) and time ($P<.0001$). Critically, both groups were stabilized with K-wire constructs instead of compression screws, and nonrigid fixation may have affected these results. On subgroup analysis of proximal pole nonunions, union was 69% (11 out of 16) for NVBG and 91% (19 out of 21) for VBG, but this was not significant ($P = .09$).

Variability of fixation and AVN assessment in these studies complicates discernment of the role of AVN in healing potential. Consequently, the necessity of VBG to achieve higher union rates or shorter time to union in patients with AVN remains unverified.

Other Factors

Prior failed surgery, proximal pole fracture location, fracture instability, humpback deformity, DISI, and proximal pole fragmentation have all been implicated as predictors of treatment failure that might support VBG.[23,27,29]

In a series of 48 SNUs treated with 1,2 ICSRA and either screw or K-wire fixation, Chang and colleagues[27] highlighted that 9 of 14 failures presented with DISI and/or humpback deformity. Jones and colleagues[23] subsequently reported a significantly higher union rate and significantly shorter union time with MFC compared with 1,2 ICSRA when DISI and/or humpback deformity were present. Although these data may suggest MFC may be indicated rather than other VBG techniques for SNU with humpback deformity, there is no evidence that VBG produces superior results to NVBG in this population.

Proximal pole fragment size is variably described (see Tables 1, 2, 4, 5) in the literature, with some investigators defining the proximal pole as the proximal fifth rather than proximal third.[5,66,67] In other studies, proximal fragment size has been reported as a percentage or ratio of the entire scaphoid according to PA radiographic or CT measurements respectively.[29,57,58] However, the authors were unable to identify large studies or meta-analyses that assessed the effect of proximal fragment size on union in NVBG versus VBG.

Previous failed surgery may also predict which patients may benefit from VBG, either from improved healing rates or time. However, there is a paucity of objective data on the impact of this factor on NVBG versus VBG outcomes.

In addition, variable instrumentation may be a considerable confounder of outcomes. Internal rigid fixation of fracture fragments is considered important for bone healing, and there is wide support for compression screw fixation.[4] K-wires may not ensure stability because of a lack of compression and loosening potential, and may confound healing rates.[68] Other investigators[69] have raised concerns that screw fixation may disrupt vascular inflow from vascularized grafts, and suggested that different fixation methods may be indicated for different graft techniques.

KEY/OPEN QUESTIONS

- Is there a diagnostic method to accurately predict vascularity (eg, ischemia/AVN/infarction)?
- Does proximal or distal pole vascularity predict healing potential?
- Can a histologically verified avascular or infarcted proximal pole heal with provision of fresh autogenous bone by creeping substitution from a well-vascularized distal pole?

- If so, does the distal pole's potential as an "engine" for healing degrade with time?
- Is the creeping substitution necessary for proximal pole healing enhanced by provision of a de novo vascular supply compared with that provided by the native distal pole?

DISCUSSION

In clinical practice, many hand surgeons argue that VBG is indicated in cases of proximal pole AVN or prior failed surgery. However, current evidence does not support improved union rates for VBG compared with traditional NVBG techniques for AVN. Analyses are complicated by ill-defined parameters for AVN diagnosis and confounded by patient and systemic factors. Consequently, bone graft choice for SNU treatment is widely debated in hand and wrist surgery.

There is no consensus on which modality best predicts proximal pole vascularity. Some investigators have reported a lack of agreement between punctate bleeding and histology,[7,38] likely because punctate bleeding is a subjective assessment with potential for inter-rater and intrarater variability.[70] Only 1 identified study, by Bervian and colleagues,[36] reported a significant correlation ($P<.05$) between punctate bleeding and histology in 19 SNUs, but biopsy specimens were not graded quantitatively.

Animal model and basic science studies comparing histology and unenhanced T_1-weighted/T_2-weighted MRI have shown that low signal intensity is not always predictive of AVN and can reflect a variety of histologic features that crowd out or decrease bone marrow fat, including fat necrosis/lipolysis (AVN), unspecified inflammatory infiltration, and fibrocytic and osseous repair.[71,72] Signal intensity changes may therefore be sensitive but not specific for histologic AVN, which may create confusion on the proportion of patients with AVN versus ischemia (compromised but not absent vascularity) in studies reporting outcomes for supposed AVN.

It is intuitive that histology would be the most objective and reproducible method to evaluate the vascular status of the scaphoid.[38,70,73,74] However, random biopsy cannot sample the totality of the scaphoid fracture fragment, and patchy patterns of AVN containing viable and dead osteocytes are frequently present side by side.[70,75,76] Techniques that use subtotal curettage of the proximal and distal poles may produce a more comprehensive evaluation of proximal pole viability.[38] Besides blood supply and stability, bone structure and biology are key factors of SNU healing and are linked to microarchitecture.[73]

Histology alone is often limited to a few parameters and may be insufficient to analyze bone remodeling.[77] Immunohistochemical studies may therefore play a role.

Schmidle and colleagues[78] compared proximal pole features defined by light and scanning electron microscopy with semiquantitative assessment of bone morphology on two-dimensional (2D) CT and fracture line location on three-dimensional (3D) CT reconstructions in 29 SNUs. Although Bervian and colleagues[36] reported no correlation between qualitative grading of histology and CT radiodensity, Schmidle and colleagues[78] found a significant correlation between histologic viability and 2D CT quantification of trabecular structure ($P<.001$) and bony fragmentation ($P = .036$). The semiquantitative assessment and more precise (0.0625 mm) CT slice algorithm used by Schmidle and colleagues[78] may explain the difference in results. The investigators suggested that fragmentation predicts the worst bone healing capacity at the proximal fragment and that vascularized osteochondral replacement may be indicated in such cases. Proximal pole fracture location relative to the scapholunate ligament on 3D CT reconstruction also significantly correlated with histologic viability ($P = .036$). CT imaging may therefore offer an improved assessment of proximal pole vascularity and healing potential given that histologic assessment cannot be performed preoperatively.

Recent studies also suggest that proximal pole vascularity may not be of preeminent prognostic potential. Rancy and colleagues[38] reported that unenhanced MRI and punctate bleeding did not agree with each other or with histologic quantification of vascularity, despite confirmed AVN in 44% (14 out of 32 SNUs). Furthermore, with thorough debridement of necrotic bone, NVBG, and rigid screw fixation, none of these variables correlated with 97% (34 out of 35) union at an average of 12 weeks (range, 6–38 weeks). These findings imply that proximal pole vascular status may be unimportant if necrotic and infarcted bone is removed and replaced by fresh autogenous bone and screw compression.

In 1999, Kulkarni and colleagues[79] observed with MRI that preserved distal fragment vascularity in 46 acute fractures facilitated advancing revascularization of proximal fragments. This healing occurs by so-called creeping substitution, involving gradual vascular ingrowth, resorption, and replacement of necrotic bone with revascularization. The process depends on the mechanical and vascular environment, particularly the vascularization of the host bed.[2] Hence,

the distal pole may be the engine for creeping substitution.

These observations agree with conclusions from a 2018 histologic and immunohistochemical study by Schmidle and colleagues,[80] who found no correlation between proximal fragment histologic viability and time from fracture ($r = 0.008$, $P = .969$), with proximal fragment viability being poor early on and remaining so. However, distal fragment viability significantly diminished with increasing time from fracture ($r = -0.427$, $P = .026$). Distal pole vascularity may therefore be a crucial prognostic factor in SNU healing. Techniques that mechanically excavate necrotic bone and replace it with viable autograft as healthy scaffolding for creeping substitution may have an advantage in healing potential, and this principle may underlie the success of several recent NVBG series.

VBG applies additional biological principles to achieve healing. Sunagawa and colleagues[81] used a canine model to show that VBG provides significantly increased bone blood flow and higher levels of osteoid-covered and osteoblast-covered trabecular surfaces compared with NVBG in surgically induced proximal pole AVN. Thus, VBG uses de novo vascularity to enhance creeping substitution of in situ necrotic bone. Whether this technique produces increased union rates or decreased time to union compared with cavitation and NVBG was not studied. Furthermore, VBG is technically demanding, costly, requires increased OR time and resources, and is has the risk of donor-site morbidity.[27,69,82] Although VBG may be beneficial in a select group of SNUs, these specific indications have yet to be substantiated.

SUMMARY AND RECOMMENDATIONS

Several factors are purported to negatively affect SNU healing after NVBG and have been recommended as indications for VBG. However, there is no evidence to support absolute indications for VBG in these cases. A growing body of evidence suggests that histologically defined proximal pole AVN can be successfully treated with cavitation of necrotic bone, NVBG, and rigid screw fixation. The authors recommend standardized reporting of proximal and distal pole vascularity, vascular assessment modality (preferably histologic quantification of necrosis or CT trabecular structure), proximal fragment size, structural defects, and fixation methods in future studies comparing reconstructive techniques. These considerations will help better define which SNUs may benefit from vascularized rather than nonvascularized grafting.

REFERENCES

1. Russe O. Fracture of the carpal navicular. Diagnosis, non-operative treatment, and operative treatment. J Bone Joint Surg Am 1960;42:759–68.

2. Büchler U, Nagy L. The issue of vascularity in fractures and nonunion of the scaphoid. J Hand Surg Br 1995;20:726–35.

3. Krimmer H. Management of acute fractures and nonunions of the proximal pole of the scaphoid. J Hand Surg Br 2002;27(3):245–8.

4. Herbert TJ, Fisher WE. Management of the fractured scaphoid using a new bone screw. J Bone Joint Surg Br 1984;66(1):114–23.

5. Steinmann SP, Adams JE. Scaphoid fractures and nonunions: diagnosis and treatment. J Orthop Sci 2006;11(4):424–31.

6. Kim J, Park JW, Chung J, et al. Non-vascularized iliac bone grafting for scaphoid nonunion with avascular necrosis. J Hand Surg Eur Vol 2018;43(1):24–31.

7. Green DP. The effect of avascular necrosis on Russe bone grafting for scaphoid nonunion. J Hand Surg Am 1985;10:597–605.

8. Robbins RR, Ridge O, Carter PR. Iliac crest bone grafting and Herbert screw fixation of nonunions of the scaphoid with avascular proximal poles. J Hand Surg Am 1995;20:818–31.

9. Günal I, Ozcelik A, Gokturk E, et al. Correlation of magnetic resonance imaging and intraoperative punctate bleeding to assess the vascularity of scaphoid nonunion. Arch Orthop Trauma Surg 1999;119:285–7.

10. Megerle K, Worg H, Christopoulos G, et al. Gadolinium-enhanced preoperative MRI scans as a prognostic parameter in scaphoid nonunion. J Hand Surg Eur Vol 2011;36:23–8.

11. Stark HH, Rickard TA, Zemel NP, et al. Treatment of ununited fractures of the scaphoid by iliac bone grafts and Kirschner-wire fixation. J Bone Joint Surg Am 1988;70(7):982–91.

12. Fernandez DL. Anterior bone grafting and conventional lag screw fixation to treat scaphoid nonunions. J Hand Surg Am 1990;15(1):140–7.

13. Finsen V, Hofstad M, Haugan H. Most scaphoid nonunions heal with bone chip grafting and Kirschner-wire fixation. Thirty-nine patients reviewed 10 years after operation. Injury 2006;37(9):854–9.

14. Dustmann M, Bajinski R, Tripp A, et al. A modified Matti-Russe technique of grafting scaphoid nonunions. Arch Orthop Trauma Surg 2017;137(6):867–73.

15. Buijze GA, Ochtman L, Ring D. Management of scaphoid nonunion. J Hand Surg Am 2012;37(5):1095–100.

16. Hovius SE, de Jong T. Bone grafts for scaphoid nonunion: an overview. Hand Surg 2015;20(2):222–7.

17. Pinder RM, Brkljac M, Rix L, et al. Treatment of scaphoid nonunion: a systematic review of the existing evidence. J Hand Surg Am 2015;40:1797–805.

18. Zaidemberg C, Siebert JW, Angrigiani C. A new vascularized bone graft for scaphoid nonunion. J Hand Surg Am 1991;16:474–8.

19. Kuhlmann JN, Mimoun M, Boabighi A, et al. Vascularized bone graft pedicled on the volar carpal artery for non-union of the scaphoid. J Hand Surg Br 1987;12(2):203–10.

20. Mathoulin C, Haerle M. Vascularized bone graft from the palmar carpal artery for treatment of scaphoid nonunion. J Hand Surg Br 1998;23(3):318–23.

21. Pechlaner S, Hussl H, Künzel KH. Alternative surgical method in pseudarthroses of the scaphoid bone. Prospective study. Handchir Mikrochir Plast Chir 1987;19(6):302–5.

22. Doi K, Oda T, Soo-Heong T, et al. Free vascularized bone graft for nonunion of the scaphoid. J Hand Surg Am 2000;25(3):507–19.

23. Jones DB Jr, Burger H, Bishop AT, et al. Treatment of scaphoid waist nonunions with an avascular proximal pole and carpal collapse. A comparison of two vascularized bone grafts. J Bone Joint Surg Am 2008;90:2616–25.

24. Ribak S, Medina CE, Mattar R Jr, et al. Treatment of scaphoid nonunion with vascularised and nonvascularised dorsal bone grafting from the distal radius. Int Orthop 2010;34:683–8.

25. Jones DB Jr, Rhee PC, Shin AY. Vascularized bone grafts for scaphoid nonunions. J Hand Surg Am 2012;37(5):1090–4.

26. Ferguson DO, Shanbhag V, Hedley H, et al. Scaphoid fracture non-union: a systematic review of surgical treatment using bone graft. J Hand Surg Eur Vol 2016;41:492–500.

27. Chang MA, Bishop AT, Moran SL, et al. The outcomes and complications of 1,2-intercompartmental supraretinacular artery pedicled vascularized bone grafting of scaphoid nonunions. J Hand Surg Am 2006;31(3):387–96.

28. Al-Jabri T, Mannan A, Giannoudis P. The use of the free vascularised bone graft for nonunion of the scaphoid: a systematic review. J Orthop Surg Res 2014;9:21.

29. Pulos N, Kollitz KM, Bishop AT, et al. Free vascularized medial femoral condyle bone graft after failed scaphoid nonunion surgery. J Bone Joint Surg Am 2018;100(16):1379–86.

30. Merrell GA, Wolfe SW, Slade JF 3rd. Treatment of scaphoid nonunions: quantitative meta-analysis of the literature. J Hand Surg Am 2002;27:685–91.

31. Braga-Silva J, Peruchi FM, Moschen GM, et al. A comparison of the use of distal radius vascularised bone graft and non-vascularised iliac crest bone graft in the treatment of non-union of scaphoid fractures. J Hand Surg Eur Vol 2008;33(5):636–40.

32. Dailiana ZH, Zachos V, Varitimidis S, et al. Scaphoid nonunions treated with vascularised bone grafts: MRI assessment. Eur J Radiol 2004;50(3):217–24.

33. Fox MG, Gaskin CM, Chhabra AB, et al. Assessment of scaphoid viability with MRI: a reassessment of findings on unenhanced MR images. AJR Am J Roentgenol 2010;195(4):W281–6.

34. Donati OF, Zanetti M, Nagy L, et al. Is dynamic gadolinium enhancement needed in MR imaging for the preoperative assessment of scaphoidal viability in patients with scaphoid nonunion? Radiology 2011; 260(3):808–16.

35. Schmitt R, Christopoulos G, Wagner M, et al. Avascular necrosis (AVN) of the proximal fragment in scaphoid nonunion: is intravenous contrast agent necessary in MRI? Eur J Radiol 2011;77(2):222–7.

36. Bervian MR, Ribak S, Livani B. Scaphoid fracture nonunion: correlation of radiographic imaging, proximal fragment histologic viability evaluation, and estimation of viability at surgery: diagnosis of scaphoid pseudarthrosis. Int Orthop 2015;39(1): 67–72.

37. Dawson JS, Martel AL, Davis TR. Scaphoid blood flow and acute fracture healing. A dynamic MRI study with enhancement with gadolinium. J Bone Joint Surg Br 2001;83(6):809–14.

38. Rancy SK, Swanstrom MM, DiCarlo EF, et al, Scaphoid Nonunion Consortium. Success of scaphoid nonunion surgery is independent of proximal pole vascularity. J Hand Surg Eur Vol 2018; 43(1):32–40.

39. Stark A, Broström LA, Svartengren G. Scaphoid nonunion treated with the Matti-Russe technique. Long-term results. Clin Orthop Relat Res 1987;(214):175–80.

40. Warren-Smith CD, Barton NJ. Non-union of the scaphoid: Russe graft vs Herbert screw. J Hand Surg Br 1988;13(1):83–6.

41. Barton NJ. Experience with scaphoid grafting. J Hand Surg Br 1997;22(2):153–60.

42. Trumble TE. Avascular necrosis after scaphoid fracture: a correlation of magnetic resonance imaging and histology. J Hand Surg Am 1990;15:557–64.

43. Morgan WJ, Breen TF, Coumas JM, et al. Role of magnetic resonance imaging in assessing factors affecting healing in scaphoid nonunions. Clin Orthop Relat Res 1997;(336):240–6.

44. Cohen MS, Jupiter JB, Fallahi K, et al. Scaphoid waist nonunion with humpback deformity treated without structural bone graft. J Hand Surg Am 2013;38(4):701–5.

45. Putnam JG, DiGiovanni RM, Mitchell SM, et al. Plate fixation with cancellous graft for scaphoid nonunion with avascular necrosis. J Hand Surg Am 2018. https://doi.org/10.1016/j.jhsa.2018.06.024.

46. Nakamura R, Horii E, Watanabe K, et al. Scaphoid non-union: factors affecting the functional outcome of open reduction and wedge grafting with Herbert screw fixation. J Hand Surg Br 1993;18(2):219–24.

47. Ritter K, Giachino AA. The treatment of pseudoarthrosis of the scaphoid by bone grafting and three methods of internal fixation. Can J Surg 2000; 43(2):118–24.

48. Matsuki H, Ishikawa J, Iwasaki N, et al. Non-vascularized bone graft with Herbert-type screw fixation for proximal pole scaphoid nonunion. J Orthop Sci 2011;16(6):749–55.

49. Sakuma M, Nakamura R, Imaeda T. Analysis of proximal fragment sclerosis and surgical outcome of scaphoid non-union by magnetic resonance imaging. J Hand Surg Br 1995;20(2):201–5.

50. Fisk GR. Carpal instability and the fractured scaphoid. Ann R Coll Surg Engl 1970;46(2):63–76.

51. Fernandez DL. A technique for anterior wedge-shaped grafts for scaphoid nonunions with carpal instability. J Hand Surg Am 1984;9(5):733–7.

52. Boyer MI, von Schroeder HP, Axelrod TS. Scaphoid nonunion with avascular necrosis of the proximal pole. Treatment with a vascularized bone graft from the dorsum of the distal radius. J Hand Surg Br 1998;23(5):686–90.

53. Steinmann SP, Bishop AT, Berger RA. Use of the 1,2 intercompartmental supraretinacular artery as a vascularized pedicle bone graft for difficult scaphoid nonunion. J Hand Surg Am 2002;27(3):391–401.

54. Straw RG, Davis TR, Dias JJ. Scaphoid nonunion: treatment with a pedicled vascularized bone graft based on the 1,2 intercompartmental supraretinacular branch of the radial artery. J Hand Surg Br 2002; 27(5):413.

55. Henry M. Collapsed scaphoid non-union with dorsal intercalated segment instability and avascular necrosis treated by vascularised wedge-shaped bone graft and fixation. J Hand Surg Eur Vol 2007; 32(2):148–54.

56. Waitayawinyu T, McCallister WV, Katolik LI, et al. Outcome after vascularized bone grafting of scaphoid nonunions with avascular necrosis. J Hand Surg Am 2009;34(3):387–94.

57. Lim TK, Kim HK, Koh KH, et al. Treatment of avascular proximal pole scaphoid nonunions with vascularized distal radius bone grafting. J Hand Surg Am 2013;38(10):1906–12.e1.

58. Morris MS, Zhu AF, Ozer K, et al. Proximal pole scaphoid nonunion reconstruction with 1,2 Intercompartmental supraretinacular artery vascularized graft and compression screw fixation. J Hand Surg Am 2018;43(8):770.e1–8.

59. Dailiana ZH, Malizos KN, Zachos V, et al. Vascularized bone grafts from the palmar radius for the treatment of waist nonunions of the scaphoid. J Hand Surg Am 2006;31(3):397–404.

60. Gras M, Mathoulin C. Vascularized bone graft pedicled on the volar carpal artery from the volar distal

radius as primary procedure for scaphoid non-union. Orthop Traumatol Surg Res 2011;97(8): 800–6.

61. Gabl M, Reinhart C, Lutz M, et al. Vascularized bone graft from the iliac crest for the treatment of nonunion of the proximal part of the scaphoid with an avascular fragment. J Bone Joint Surg Am 1999;81(10):1414–28.

62. Harpf C, Gabl M, Reinhart C, et al. Small free vascularized iliac crest bone grafts in reconstruction of the scaphoid bone: a retrospective study in 60 cases. Plast Reconstr Surg 2001;108(3):664–74.

63. Arora R, Lutz M, Zimmermann R, et al. Free vascularised iliac bone graft for recalcitrant avascular nonunion of the scaphoid. J Bone Joint Surg Br 2010;92(2):224–9.

64. Hirche C, Xiong L, Heffinger C, et al. Vascularized versus non-vascularized bone grafts in the treatment of scaphoid non-union. J Orthop Surg (Hong Kong) 2017;25(1). 2309499016684291.

65. Munk B, Larsen CF. Bone grafting the scaphoid nonunion: a systematic review of 147 publications including 5,246 cases of scaphoid nonunion. Acta Orthop Scand 2004;75(5):618–29.

66. Gelberman RH, Menon J. The vascularity of the scaphoid bone. J Hand Surg Am 1980;5(5):508–13.

67. Eastley N, Singh H, Dias JJ, et al. Union rates after proximal scaphoid fractures; meta-analyses and review of available evidence. J Hand Surg Eur Vol 2013;38(8):888–97.

68. Pao VS, Chang J. Scaphoid nonunion: diagnosis and treatment. Plast Reconstr Surg 2003;112(6): 1666–76 [quiz: 1677]; [discussion: 1678–9].

69. Alluri RK, Yin C, Iorio ML, et al. A critical appraisal of vascularized bone grafting for scaphoid nonunion. J Wrist Surg 2017;6(3):251–7.

70. Larribe M, Gay A, Freire V, et al. Usefulness of dynamic contrast-enhanced MRI in the evaluation of the viability of acute scaphoid fracture. Skeletal Radiol 2014;43(12):1697–703.

71. Simmons DJ, Daum WJ, Totty W, et al. Correlation of MRI images with histology in avascular necrosis in the hip. A preliminary study. J Arthroplasty 1989; 4(1):7–14.

72. Brody AS, Strong M, Babikian G, et al. Avascular necrosis: early MR imaging and histologic findings in a canine model. AJR Am J Roentgenol 1991;157(2): 341–5.

73. Qu G, von Schroeder HP. Trabecular microstructure at the human scaphoid nonunion. J Hand Surg 2008;33(5):650–5.

74. Rein S, Hanisch U, Rammelt S, et al. Histopathological, radiological and clinical aspects of the temporal assignment of scaphoid non-union. Arch Orthop Trauma Surg 2010;130(10):1243–50.

75. Urban MA, Green DP, Aufdemorte TB. The patchy configuration of scaphoid avascular necrosis. J Hand Surg Am 1993;18(4):669–74.

76. Cerezal L, Abascal F, Canga A, et al. Usefulness of gadolinium-enhanced MR imaging in the evaluation of the vascularity of scaphoid nonunions. AJR Am J Roentgenol 2000;174(1):141–9.

77. Rein S, Hanisch U, Schaller HE, et al. Evaluation of bone remodeling in regard to the age of scaphoid non-unions. World J Orthop 2016;7(7):418–25.

78. Schmidle G, Ebner HL, Klauser AS, et al. Correlation of CT imaging and histology to guide bone graft selection in scaphoid non-union surgery. Arch Orthop Trauma Surg 2018. https://doi.org/10.1007/s00402-018-2983-0.

79. Kulkarni RW, Wollstein R, Tayar R, et al. Patterns of healing of scaphoid fractures. The importance of vascularity. J Bone Joint Surg Br 1999;81(1):85–90.

80. Schmidle G, Ebner HL, Klima G, et al. Time-dependent changes in bone healing capacity of scaphoid fractures and non-unions. J Anat 2018;232(6): 908–18.

81. Sunagawa T, Bishop AT, Muramatsu K. Role of conventional and vascularized bone grafts in scaphoid nonunion with avascular necrosis: a canine experimental study. J Hand Surg Am 2000;25(5):849–59.

82. Alluri RK, Yin C, Iorio ML, et al. Vascularized bone grafting in scaphoid nonunion: a review of patient-centered outcomes. Hand (N Y) 2017;12(2):127–34.

Long-Term Outcomes of Vascularized Trochlear Flaps for Scaphoid Proximal Pole Reconstruction

Mitchell A. Pet, MD[a], James P. Higgins, MD[b],*

KEYWORDS

- Medial femoral trochlea • Proximal pole scaphoid nonunion • Osteochondral free flap
- Vascularized cartilage transfer • Patient-reported outcomes

KEY POINTS

- Medial femoral trochlea osteochondral flap reconstruction of the scaphoid's proximal pole union is offered to young patients as an alternative to conventional wrist salvage procedures.
- Two publications provide most reported outcomes information available. One describes recipient site outcomes, and the other addresses donor site morbidity.
- This study provides a brief update of clinical, radiographic, and patient-reported outcomes seen in the subset of our patients with greater than 3 years of postoperative follow-up.
- The currently available outcomes information suggests that MFT reconstruction for proximal pole scaphoid nonunion can restore radiocarpal anatomy, prevent progressive carpal collapse, improve function, and relieve pain without causing wrist stiffness, weakness, or excessive donor site morbidity in the short and medium term.
- Additional follow-up and application of expanded outcomes measures are necessary to comprehensively evaluate long-term outcomes in this population.

INTRODUCTION

Revision surgery for proximal pole scaphoid nonunion is technically challenging. Contributing factors may include bone loss from prior fixation attempts, and fragmentation or poor perfusion of the scaphoid's proximal pole. In older patients with low functional demand, salvage operations, such as proximal row carpectomy or four corner fusion, obviate scaphoid reconstruction, and can produce satisfactory results.[1] In younger patients, these salvage operations may fail to meet their high functional demands and eventually lead to radiocarpal arthritis.[2] For this reason, there has been increasing interest in reconstruction of the proximal scaphoid. Alternative means of restoring wrist anatomy and kinematics have been suggested, including prosthetic arthroplasty,[3] non-vascularized osteochondral autografting,[4] and vascularized osteochondral flap reconstruction.[5–7]

One such method of scaphoid restoration is the use of the medial femoral trochlea (MFT) flap. The MFT is an osteochondral free flap harvested from a non–weight bearing portion of the ipsilateral patellofemoral joint, which is similar in shape to the scaphoid proximal pole.[8] The osteochondral segment is vascularized by the transverse branch

Disclosure: The authors have no conflicts of interest and there was no funding for this article.
[a] Plastic and Reconstructive Surgery Center, Center for Advanced Medicine, 4921 Parkview Place, Suite G, Floor 6, St. Louis, MO 63110, USA; [b] Curtis National Hand Center, MedStar Union Memorial Hospital, 3333 North Calvert Street, JPB Mezzanine, M50, Baltimore, MD 21208, USA
* Corresponding author.
E-mail address: jameshiggins10@hotmail.com

Hand Clin 35 (2019) 345–352
https://doi.org/10.1016/j.hcl.2019.03.006

of the descending geniculate artery,[7] which descends parallel to the medial column of the femur, directly beneath the vastus medialis. The use of this bone for proximal pole reconstruction involves resection of the proximal half of the scaphoid, insertion of the MFT flap to replace the proximal pole of the scaphoid, and then establishment of blood flow to the flap via anastomosis into the radial artery system. Although the procedure requires microsurgery, it facilitates ease of fixation by providing a large, high-quality segment of bone to secure at the waist-level osteosynthesis site. In a porcine survival study of this procedure, vascularized osteochondral flaps demonstrated superior cartilage retention compared with non-vascularized analogous grafts attributable to the dense vascular supply.[9]

This surgical intervention is designed to restore the shape of the proximal pole, prevent progressive carpal collapse, improve function, and relieve pain. As such, a complete outcomes assessment must include clinical, radiographic, and patient-reported outcomes (PROs).

SURGICAL TECHNIQUE

Our surgical technique for MFT reconstruction of the proximal scaphoid has been previously published.[7] Briefly, a dorsal approach is made to the carpus and the wrist is flexed to expose the proximal pole nonunion. Any existing hardware is removed, and then the proximal pole of the scaphoid including the nonunited segment is resected. The scaphoid osteotomy for proximal pole resection is oblique with respect to axis of the bone, and is illustrated in **Fig. 1**. The obliquity of the osteotomy creates a fresh cut surface, which parallels the scaphoid facet, and allows preservation of the most distal portion of the scapholunate interosseous ligament. The MFT flap is then harvested from the ipsilateral knee, and trimmed to fit the carpal defect. The osteochondral flap is inserted into the carpal defect and provisional fixation is achieved with K-wires. Osteosynthesis is then achieved using an anterograde cannulated headless compression screw. Microsurgical anastomosis (end-to-side

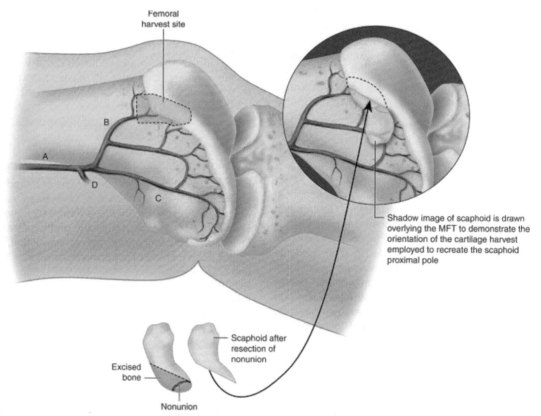

Fig. 1. Representation of MFT and the planned portion of reconstructed proximal scaphoid. Portion of MFT harvested to provide vascularized osteocartilaginous reconstruction of the proximal scaphoid. A, descending geniculate artery. B, transverse branch. C, longitudinal branch. D, superiomedial geniculate artery. (*From* Bürger HK, Windhofer C, Gaggl AJ, et al. Vascularized medial femoral trochlea osteocartilaginous flap reconstruction of proximal pole scaphoid nonunions. J Hand Surg Am 2013;38(4):694; and the Curtis National Hand Center, Baltimore, MD; with permission.)

artery, end-to-end vein) is then performed into the radial artery system. A brief case report demonstrating typical preoperative, intraoperative, and postoperative radiographs is seen in **Fig. 2**.

REVIEW OF EXISTING LITERATURE
Recipient Site

The existing literature surrounding outcomes of MFT flap reconstruction for proximal scaphoid nonunion is limited. The largest series of reconstructed scaphoid outcomes was published in 2013, and reflects the early combined experience of Dr Heinz Bürger in Austria, and The Curtis National Hand Center in Baltimore.[5] In this publication, a series of 16 reconstructed scaphoids was documented, with a minimum follow-up of 6 months and a mean follow-up of 14 months. Union was achieved in 15 patients. Improvement in wrist pain was documented in all patients, with 12 experiencing complete pain relief. Postoperative wrist range of motion averaged 46° of extension, and 44° of flexion, which was nearly identical to preoperative measurements. Pronation, supination, and digital range of motion were unaffected. Radiographic follow-up revealed a scapholunate angle of 52° before surgery and 49° after surgery.

We are only aware of one additional group that has published outcomes of MFT-based reconstructive surgery. In 2017, Tremp and colleagues[10] documented two cases of MFT harvest; one for reconstruction of the proximal scaphoid pole, and one for reconstruction of the talus. Bony union was achieved in each case, and after 36 months of follow-up, their scaphoid reconstruction patient reported minimal wrist pain (visual analogue scale = 2), and maintained a 50° of wrist extension and 20° degrees of wrist flexion (60° extension and 20° flexion preoperatively).

Donor Site

A systematic review of donor site morbidity for vascularized flaps from the distal femur was published by Giladi and colleagues[11] in 2018. Although they were able to identify 45 papers reporting on this topic, only three of the papers (reporting 50 unique patients) discuss the MFT, whereas the remainder address the medial femoral condyle flap. The largest of these three available studies was published in 2016.[12] This series consisted of 45 patients, 30 who had undergone MFT harvest for scaphoid reconstruction, and 15 who had reconstruction of the lunate for advanced Kienböck disease. Because the donor site harvest technique is the same for both carpal reconstructive techniques, combining these two groups for the purpose of evaluating donor site study is reasonable.

Minimum follow-up in the series was 9 months (mean, 27 months), and 81% of eligible patients participated in the study. No early postoperative donor site complications (ie, cellulitis, abscess, hematoma, iatrogenic fracture, or wound dehiscence) were encountered. Follow-up examination revealed a stable knee in all patients and no deficits in range of motion. MRI in all of those examined (35 patients) revealed no pathologic changes. Average duration of postoperative pain was just over 2 months, and 58% underwent postoperative physical therapy. Patients reported returning to normal knee function approximately 3 months after surgery. At last follow-up, four patients had continuous knee pain throughout the day, and 10 patients endorsed intermittent knee pain. The average International Knee Documentation Committee score in this series was 96, the average Western Ontario and McMaster University (WOMAC) score was at 94% (corresponding to 6% disability). Patient satisfaction with surgery was rated highly on a Likert scale, and 98% of patients said they would have the same surgery again.

Three additional patients were reported by the same collaborators in a subsequent series on MFT reconstruction of the lunate.[13] Each of these patients had intermittent discomfort for 1 to 3 months postoperatively, followed by complete resolution. The series by Tremp and colleagues[10] offers little information on their series of two patients who underwent MFT harvest, but it is noted that no donor site complications were encountered.

UPDATE ON OUR CENTER'S MIDTERM OUTCOMES DATA

As of January 2018, we had performed MFT reconstruction of the proximal pole of the scaphoid for 41 patients at the Curtis National Hand Center. Within our series of 41 patients, 19 underwent MFT reconstruction of the scaphoid greater than 3 years ago. Among these patients, complete postoperative clinical and radiographic follow-up data were available for 10 patients (53%). Mean follow-up for this subgroup of 10 patients was 4.1 years (range, 3–6 years), and mean age at surgery was 21.5 years (range, 16–27 years). Seven of the 10 patients were male, and six injuries were dominant-sided. Each patient underwent MFT reconstruction for the indication of proximal pole scaphoid nonunion status post unsuccessful open reduction and internal fixation.

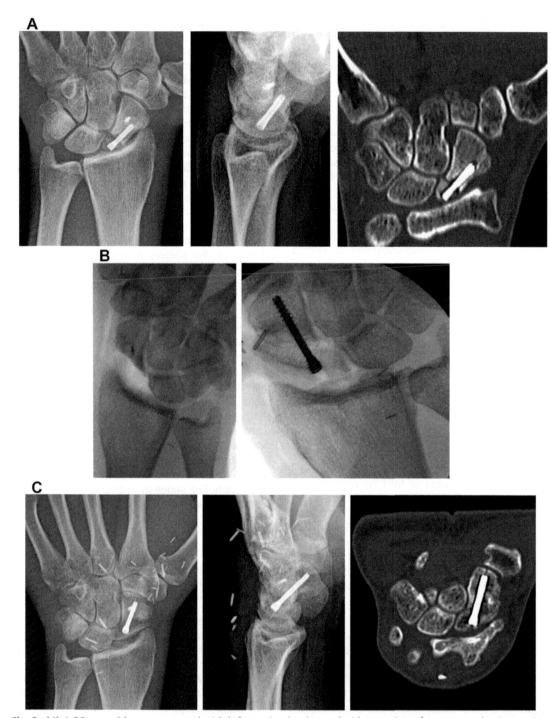

Fig. 2. (*A*) A 26-year-old man presented with left proximal pole scaphoid nonunion after open reduction and internal fixation with a cannulated headless compression screw. (*B*) Based on the patient's young age and preserved scaphoid facet, he elected to pursue medial femoral trochlea flap reconstruction of the scaphoid's proximal pole. This figure demonstrates intraoperative posteroanterior radiographs of the wrist after proximal pole excision (*left*), and replacement with the osteochondral flap, which is fixated using a cannulated headless compression screw (*right*). (*C*) Late postoperative posteroanterior and lateral radiographs in addition to a representative coronal plane computed tomography scan image demonstrate union of the distal scaphoid pole and osteochondral segment. A neutral lunate posture and normal scapholunate angle are evident, and no scapholunate diastasis is noted.

Clinical Outcomes

In this cohort, postoperative flexion/extension was 42.8°/42.3° (69%/63% of contralateral), and radial/ulnar deviation was 10.7°/31° (50%/74% of contralateral). Grip strength averaged 32.2 kg (81% of contralateral). These parameters fall short of the normal contralateral side, but this amount of wrist motion is functional for most activities.[14,15]

The lone recipient site complication in this group was an instance of wound dehiscence requiring debridement and secondary closure. Additionally, one patient experienced ongoing knee pain, which was eventually successfully treated with arthroscopic debridement.

Radiographic Outcomes

All 10 patients went on to union between the distal scaphoid and osteochondral segment, as demonstrated by computed tomography scan at 3 months postoperatively. To evaluate carpal alignment and longitudinal carpal collapse, respectively, we measured the radiolunate (RL) angle and carpal height ratio (carpal height divided by third metacarpal length).[16] Although we have previously reported carpal alignment in terms of scapholunate angle,[7] we currently favor these radiographic parameters because neither is affected by difficulties in delineating the axis of a collapsed or reconstructed scaphoid.

In this cohort, RL angle was found to be −6.3° (slight dorsal tilt) at a mean of 4.1 years (range, 3–6 years). This is a near-neutral posture slightly better than the preoperative measurement of −16.9[a] and lies well within the normal range of +15° to −15°.[17] We attribute this normal carpal alignment to preservation of the distal most portion of the scapholunate interosseous ligament, along with the achievement of bony scaphoid union with intentional "overstuffing" of the resection cavity.[18]

Carpal height ratio in this cohort was found to be 0.50 at the same interval of follow-up. This near-normal[16] value is slightly improved from the preoperative measurement of 0.48[b], reflecting that carpal collapse was halted during the follow-up period.

The final, and perhaps most important, radiographic outcome of this procedure is the occurrence of radioscaphoid arthritis. In our cohort of 10 patients, one showed evidence of progression of radioscaphoid arthritis (Watson stage II). This patient demonstrated the most abnormal postoperative RL angle (−29°), which deteriorated from a preoperative value of −11°. In this patient, it is likely that we either failed to preserve the distal aspect of the dorsal scapholunate ligament, failed to adequately overstuff the proximal pole resection cavity, or both. However, despite this radiographic outcome, this patient had a disabilities of the arm, shoulder, and hand (DASH) score of 0 at 3.2 years after surgery.

Patient-Reported Outcomes

For specific outcomes assessment of the wrist, we have relied on the DASH score administered preoperatively and postoperatively. In this group of 10 patients, the average postoperative DASH score was 7.5 (range, 0–18), which is improved from a preoperative mean of 24[c] (range, 2–44) at a mean of 4 years (range, 3.1–5.0 years). Although statistical comparison cannot be responsibly applied to this small cohort, these values are put in some context by noting that the minimal clinically important difference for the DASH score is 10.[19]

Although the observed improvements in wrist function are encouraging, one also has to consider the potential for donor site morbidity in a previously normal knee. We have followed donor site morbidity at the knee using the Knee Injury and Osteoarthritis Outcome Score (KOOS) questionnaire, and its derivative, the WOMAC Osteoarthritis Index. The KOOS scale is a detailed 42-item questionnaire with five subscales specifically querying the patient experience as it relates to knee pain, symptoms, activities of daily living (ADL), sports and recreation, and quality of life.[20] The WOMAC is a patient-reported measure of overall knee health combining pain, stiffness, and functional limitation.[21,22] Each scale is measured from 0 (no function) to 100 (ideal function).

In our cohort of 10 patients at a mean of 4 years (range, 3.1–5.0 years), the mean KOOS pain score was 91, KOOS symptoms was 87, KOOS ADL was 95, KOOS sports and recreation was 80, and KOOS quality of life was 85. The mean WOMAC score was 94. Because these PRO scales may be unfamiliar to hand surgeons, some context is helpful. In 2016, Muller and colleagues[23] defined

---

[a] Preoperative RL angle values only available in 7 of 10 patients.

[b] Preoperative carpal height ratio values only available in 7 of 10 patients.

[c] Preoperative DASH score available in 8 of 10 patients.

the Patient Acceptable Symptom State (PASS) thresholds for the KOOS subscales. The PASS threshold describes a minimum cutoff point at which most of the population "feels well" in a given PRO domain. In our population, postoperative scores remained well above the PASS thresholds for the International Knee Documentation Committee and all KOOS subscales. The only exception to this was the KOOS ADL subscale, which is known to have the lowest sensitivity for patient wellness. It is reasonable to expect that most patients will feel "well" with respect to knee function after MFT harvest.

DISCUSSION

The concept of proximal scaphoid excision and replacement in the setting of nonunion was described almost 20 years ago. In 1989, Carter and colleagues[24] published a series of eight patients who underwent proximal pole replacement with nonvascularized scaphoid allograft. They observed reliable union occurring between 6 and 12 months postoperatively, demonstrated good results in 75% of patients at a mean of 17 months. Two patients developed graft collapse at mid-term follow-up. Additionally, late biopsy of the graft in two cases revealed abnormal-appearing cartilage, with few viable chondrocytes and no viable osteocytes at the proximal extent of the graft. This is cause for some concern that these allografts may not ultimately be a viable long-term solution for reconstruction of the proximal pole.

Recognizing that the allogenic nature of this graft reconstruction may be disadvantageous, Sandow[4] developed a technique of costo-osteochondral autograft reconstruction of the scaphoid proximal pole. Outcomes for 47 patients undergoing this reconstruction have been documented, with a median follow-up of 15 months. Because there is only a small bony segment included in this largely chondral autograft, the authors are unable to determine if union is routinely achieved. They have, however, observed no instances of graft displacement or symptomatic nonunion. Sandow[25] reported the opportunity to biopsy the cartilage grafts in four patients that underwent subsequent operative interventions at a median of 18 months after their initial grafting procedure. The biopsy demonstrated "variable survival of surface and deeper chondrocytes with changes in the articulating surface suggestive of adaptive metaplasia."[25] As with the other techniques discussed in this article, long-term outcomes data are lacking, and few conclusions can be made regarding potential for this surgery to offer ongoing carpal integrity.

The authors believe that the use of vascularized autogenous cartilage represents an advantage over osteochondral graft reconstruction. This hypothesis has been supported by work comparing cartilage quality of vascularized osteochondral flaps and nonvascularized osteochondral grafts.[9] In this study the two different osteochondral segments were reharvested and underwent blinded histologic evaluation 6 months after transfer in a porcine model. The vascularized osteochondral flaps demonstrated superior survival, morphology, and histology compared with the nonvascularized grafts when assessed using the International Cartilage Repair Society Visual Histologic Assessment Scale. It is based on this finding that we continue to prefer proximal pole reconstruction with vascularized autogenous tissue.

The clinical follow-up available in our series of MFT flaps is best described as short and intermediate term. For the purposes of this solicited review, we have outlined the available studies and added a small cohort of our patients with follow-up data exceeding 3 years in duration. A more complete report on the larger cohort of patients from our institution is currently under peer review and will provide additional insight into the value of this operation for scaphoid nonunion patients. Meticulous ongoing data collection will continue to assess the procedure's value over decades of follow-up in these young patients. Given the limitations of current data and experience available, some early conclusions can be provided and are summarized herein.

Recipient Site

Although the series is small, the study by Bürger and colleagues[7] suggests that the rate of union for scaphoid reconstruction using the MFT flap is high[7] when performed in a subset of patients with particularly challenging recalcitrant nonunions and small and/or fragmented proximal poles. Additionally, pain relief and motion preservation are demonstrated, as is the ability of MFT reconstruction to maintain normal carpal alignment. The weaknesses of this outcomes study include its limited follow-up duration, restricted set of clinical and radiographic outcomes measures, and lack of PRO measures.

In preparing this current brief report of 10 patients with the longest available follow-up, the authors have tried to address these limitations. These results are consistent with the previous findings of reliable bony union, and stable range of motion. Furthermore, prior evidence of carpal alignment and stability is supported by our finding of normal RL angle with maintenance of carpal height. Additionally, suggestion of upper extremity functional improvement is supported by the substantial observed improvements in DASH score.

The authors believe that carpal stability is contributed to both by preservation of the most distal aspect of the scapholunate ligament and by overstuffing of the proximal pole resection cavity. Overstuffing is the practice of reconstructing the scaphoid proximal pole with an MFT flap that fits tightly into the resection cavity, and is slightly larger than the native proximal pole. This has been shown to restore normal lunate posture in a cadaveric biomechanical model after complete resection of the scapholunate ligament and secondary ligamentous scapholunate stabilizing structures.[16] Additionally, Sandow[4] has commented that restoring height of the lateral carpal column, the volar RL ligaments can be tensioned, thus preventing a mild dorsal intercalated segment instability. Our team is currently investigating the effect of scaphoid overstuffing on radiocarpal contact pressures in a cadaver model. The long-term effects of this practice require longer term follow-up on this cohort of patients.

Although one patient has demonstrated early radioscaphoid arthritis in the setting of a dorsal intercalated segment instability deformity, this patient had a follow-up DASH score of 0, which is indicative of normal function. As in other degenerative processes of the upper extremity, radiographic findings after MFT reconstruction may not always predict the patient experience. This underscores the importance of PRO measures as an essential component of MFT outcomes assessment.

Donor Site

The donor site outcomes study by Windhofer and colleagues[12] offers extensive follow-up and reported a subset of patients with PRO information.[12] Some limitations of this study are that it included patients with only 9 months of follow-up, and that the chosen PRO scales describe only aggregate knee function, which limits the ability to understand exactly how donor site morbidity may affect the lives of patients.

The current report supports the prior finding of preserved range of motion and satisfactory PRO scores after MFT harvest. By applying the KOOS PRO measure to this population, we were also able to obtain more granular data regarding postoperative knee function. At 3 years postoperatively, the areas showing some donor site morbidity are related to sports and recreation, whereas routine ADL are less affected. This domain-specific information may be helpful to patients and surgeons deciding whether or not this donor site is acceptable in a given situation.

SUMMARY

In this article, the authors review the existing literature on outcomes of the MFT flap for reconstruction of the proximal scaphoid. Additionally, we offer an up-to-date report on our 10 patients with the longest and most comprehensive follow-up available. Based on this information, we believe that there is substantial evidence suggesting that this intervention can restore radiocarpal anatomy, prevent progressive carpal collapse, improve function, and relieve pain without causing wrist stiffness, weakness, or excessive donor site morbidity in the short and medium term.

Because this is a new technique, true long-term follow-up does not yet exist. This is an important consideration because this reconstruction is specifically offered to patients in their teenage years, 20s, and 30s, who will test its longevity for decades to come. Despite this uncertainty, which is inherent to the maturation of any surgical advancement, we believe that the available data are encouraging and support ongoing investigation. As our experience grows and follow-up accrues, we will continue to monitor these patients with yearly radiographs, clinical examinations, and PRO questionnaires.

REFERENCES

1. Saltzman BM, Frank JM, Slikker W, et al. Clinical outcomes of proximal row carpectomy versus four-corner arthrodesis for post-traumatic wrist arthropathy: a systematic review. J Hand Surg Eur Vol 2015;40(5):450–7.

2. Wagner ER, Werthel J-D, Elhassan BT, et al. Proximal row carpectomy and 4-corner arthrodesis in patients younger than age 45 years. J Hand Surg 2017; 42(6):428–35.

3. Gras M, Wahegaonkar A, Mathoulin C. Treatment of avascular necrosis of the proximal pole of the scaphoid by arthroscopic resection and prosthetic semireplacement arthroplasty using the pyrocarbon adaptive proximal scaphoid implant (APSI): long-term functional outcomes. J Wrist Surg 2012; 01(02):159–64.

4. Sandow MJ. Costo-osteochondral grafts in the wrist. Tech Hand Up Extrem Surg 2001;5(3):165–72.

5. Higgins J, Burger H. Proximal scaphoid arthroplasty using the medial femoral trochlea flap. J Wrist Surg 2013;02(03):228–33.

6. Higgins JP, Bürger HK. The use of osteochondral flaps in the treatment of carpal disorders. J Hand Surg Eur Vol 2018;43(1):48–56.

7. Bürger HK, Windhofer C, Gaggl AJ, et al. Vascularized medial femoral trochlea osteocartilaginous flap reconstruction of proximal pole scaphoid nonunions. J Hand Surg Am 2013;38(4):690–700.

8. Hugon S, Koninckx A, Barbier O. Vascularized osteochondral graft from the medial femoral trochlea: anatomical study and clinical perspectives. Surg Radiol Anat 2010;32(9):817–25.

9. Higgins JP, Borumandi F, Bürger HK, et al. Nonvascularized cartilage grafts versus vascularized cartilage flaps: comparison of cartilage quality 6 months after transfer. J Hand Surg 2018;43(2):188. e1–8.

10. Tremp M, Haumer A, Wettstein R, et al. The medial femoral trochlea flap with a monitor skin island: report of two cases. Microsurgery 2016;37(5):431–5.

11. Giladi AM, Rinkinen JR, Higgins JP, et al. Donor-site morbidity of vascularized bone flaps from the distal femur: a systematic review. Plast Reconstr Surg 2018;142(3):363e–72e.

12. Windhofer C, Wong VW, Larcher L, et al. Knee donor site morbidity following harvest of medial femoral trochlea osteochondral flaps for carpal reconstruction. J Hand Surg 2016;41(5):610–4.e1.

13. Bürger HK, Windhofer C, Gaggl AJ, et al. Vascularized medial femoral trochlea osteochondral flap reconstruction of advanced Kienböck disease. J Hand Surg Am 2014;39(7):1313–22.

14. Ryu JY, Cooney WP, Askew LJ, et al. Functional ranges of motion of the wrist joint. J Hand Surg Am 1991;16(3):409–19.

15. Palmer AK, Werner FW, Murphy D, et al. Functional wrist motion: a biomechanical study. J Hand Surg Am 1985;10(1):39–46.

16. Youm Y, McMurthy RY, Flatt AE, et al. Kinematics of the wrist. I. An experimental study of radial-ulnar deviation and flexion-extension. J Bone Joint Surg Am 1978;60(4):423–31.

17. Döring A-C, Overbeek CL, Teunis T, et al. A slightly dorsally tilted lunate on MRI can be considered normal. Arch Bone Jt Surg 2016;4(4):348–52.

18. Capito AE, Higgins JP. Scaphoid overstuffing: the effects of the dimensions of scaphoid reconstruction on scapholunate alignment. J Hand Surg 2013; 38(12):2419–25.

19. Gummesson C, Atroshi I, Ekdahl C. The disabilities of the arm, shoulder and hand (DASH) outcome questionnaire: longitudinal construct validity and measuring self-rated health change after surgery. BMC Musculoskelet Disord 2003;4:11.

20. Bekkers JEJ, de Windt TS, Raijmakers NJH, et al. Validation of the knee injury and osteoarthritis outcome score (KOOS) for the treatment of focal cartilage lesions. Osteoarthritis Cartilage 2009; 17(11):1434–9.

21. Johanson NA, Liang MH, Daltroy L, et al. American Academy of Orthopaedic Surgeons lower limb outcomes assessment instruments. Reliability, validity, and sensitivity to change. J Bone Joint Surg Am 2004;86-A(5):902–9.

22. Roos EM, Klässbo M, Lohmander LS. WOMAC osteoarthritis index. Reliability, validity, and responsiveness in patients with arthroscopically assessed osteoarthritis. Western Ontario and MacMaster Universities. Scand J Rheumatol 1999;28(4):210–5.

23. Muller B, Yabroudi MA, Lynch A, et al. Defining thresholds for the patient acceptable symptom state for the IKDC subjective knee form and KOOS for patients who underwent ACL reconstruction. Am J Sports Med 2016;44(11):2820–6.

24. Carter PR, Malinin TI, Abbey PA, et al. The scaphoid allograft: a new operation for treatment of the very proximal scaphoid nonunion or for the necrotic, fragmented scaphoid proximal pole. J Hand Surg Am 1989;14(1):1–12.

25. Sandow MJ. Proximal scaphoid costo-osteochondral replacement arthroplasty. J Hand Surg Br 2016; 23(2):201–8.

Volar Radius Vascularized Bone Flaps for the Treatment of Scaphoid Nonunion

Kate Elzinga, MD[a],*, Kevin C. Chung, MD, MS[b]

KEYWORDS

- Avascular necrosis • Distal radius bone graft • Pedicled bone flap • Preiser disease
- Pronator quadratus • Scaphoid fracture • Scaphoid nonunion • Vascularized bone flap

KEY POINTS

- Volar vascularized bone flaps (VBFs) are indicated for scaphoid reconstruction for patients with scaphoid nonunion with avascular necrosis of the proximal pole and/or humpback deformity. They result in faster union rates than nonvascularized grafts.
- The volar carpal artery and pronator quadratus VBFs are most commonly used. Corticocancellous bone flaps, which impart greater structural support, are harvested and can be rotated distally into scaphoid defects.
- The pisiform VBF is covered in articular cartilage and can be used when replacement of the proximal pole of the scaphoid is required.
- The volar distal ulna VBF is less commonly used, because it requires sacrifice of the ulnar artery.

INTRODUCTION

Vascularized bone flaps (VBFs) are indicated for patients with scaphoid nonunion that is long-standing or that results in avascular necrosis (AVN) of the proximal pole of the scaphoid and for patients with Preiser disease.[1] Cortical osteocyte viability, bone mass, strength, and elastic modulus are greater compared with nonvascularized bone grafts, resulting in faster union times.[2,3] Volar VBFs are preferred over dorsal VBFs in patients with scaphoid nonunion with a humpback deformity and AVN. A volar surgical approach avoids damage to vessels entering the dorsal ridge of the scaphoid.

The goals of scaphoid nonunion treatment with a VBF are revascularization of the scaphoid, restoration of carpal alignment, and avoidance of radiographic progression of wrist arthritis (scaphoid nonunion advanced collapse [SNAC]), resulting in improvements in pain, grip, strength, and function. Range of motion cannot be reliably improved with a VBF. Reconstruction of a scaphoid nonunion with AVN using a VBF can avoid the need for salvage surgery, for example, a partial carpal fusion (4-corner fusion or lunocapitate fusion most commonly) or a proximal row carpectomy (PRC).

The VBF must have a sufficient arc of rotation and size to restore the anatomy of the scaphoid. This article reviews the surgical technique for harvest of 4 pedicled volar VBFs available for scaphoid reconstruction:

Disclosure Statement: The authors have nothing to disclose.
[a] Section of Plastic Surgery, University of Calgary, Foothills Medical Centre, Room 382, 1403 - 29 Street Northwest, Calgary, Alberta T2N 2T9, Canada; [b] Section of Plastic Surgery, The University of Michigan Medical School, 1500 East Medical Center Drive, 2130 Taubman Center, SPC 5340, Ann Arbor, MI 48109-0340, USA
* Corresponding author.
E-mail address: kate.elzinga@ahs.ca

Hand Clin 35 (2019) 353–363
https://doi.org/10.1016/j.hcl.2019.03.012

1. Volar carpal artery VBF
2. Pronator quadratus VBF
3. Volar distal ulna VBF
4. Pisiform VBF

ALTERNATIVES TO PEDICLED VOLAR VASCULARIZED BONE FLAPS

Pedicled VBFs avoid the need for a distal donor site and microsurgical anastomosis. However, the arc of rotation of pedicled flaps is limited, often requiring wrist flexion to achieve inset of the VBF. This positioning can make internal fixation of the scaphoid difficult. Free flaps permit unrestricted placement of the bone flap into the defect without constraints from the pedicle and may be necessary for large scaphoid bone defects, because the size of flap harvested from a regional pedicled site can be limited. The medial femoral condyle and trochlear flaps are the most commonly used free flaps for volar vascularized bone grafting of the carpus.[4,5] Free flaps from the iliac crest and rib can also be used.[6,7]

The medial femoral condyle is an excellent corticocancellous flap for thin patients with scaphoid defects. In obese or muscular patients, the medial femoral condyle can be more difficult to access and may have greater donor site morbidity, in particular wound healing complications. In these cases, a volar pedicled VBF from the distal radius is preferred.

PRINCIPLES OF VASCULARIZED BONE FLAPS

Intraoperative assessment of the scaphoid before VBF harvest is recommended, taking care to avoid damage to the surrounding vessels that may serve as pedicles. Exposure of the scaphoid permits debridement of sclerotic bone and fibrous tissue, assessment of proximal pole vascularity, measurement of defect size (length, width, depth), and evaluation for arthritis at the radiocarpal joint. The proximal and distal scaphoid should be debrided until healthy bleeding bone is seen. If arthritic changes are present, the operative plan should be altered accordingly. Radial styloidectomy is recommended for stage 1 SNAC, whereas salvage surgeries should be considered for SNAC stage 2 to 4 (partial or total wrist fusion, PRC).

A dorsal intercalated segmental instability (DISI) can be corrected by flexing the wrist to obtain neutral alignment of the lunate relative to the distal radius and then the lunate can be held in this position with an antegrade Kirschner wire (K wire) from the dorsal radius into the lunate. The scaphoid alignment can then be corrected and scaphoid height reestablished using joysticks in the proximal and distal scaphoid. The distal scaphoid fragment typically needs to be extended and supinated. The VBF can then be harvested with its size based on the gap between the reduced proximal and distal scaphoid fragments. A small lamina spreader can be used to help reestablish the scaphoid height and to create space for VBF insertion at the nonunion site. The VBF should be harvested 2 mm oversize to help with restoration of scaphoid stability and to account for compression when the flap is fixated. During flap harvest, an additional bone cut can be made at a 45° angle proximal to the flap so that the flap is levered out of the bone with the desired shape and without fracturing.[8]

Tourniquet use, without exsanguination of the limb, is recommended to facilitate pedicle identification and dissection. Skeletonization of the pedicle should be avoided; harvest with surrounding tissue aids with flap vascularity, in particular venous outflow. Vascular microclips and microbipolar forceps are helpful for dividing small vascular branches during flap elevation. Loupe, or less commonly microscope, magnification is essential.

INTERNAL FIXATION OF VASCULARIZED BONE FLAPS FOR SCAPHOID NONUNION

Volar VBFs can be fixated with temporary K wires (typically removal occurs 8 weeks postoperatively), retrograde headless compression screws, or volar buttress scaphoid plates depending on the flap size and the fracture pattern.[9] Rigid stability and direct bone contact are important when treating scaphoid fractures, both in acute and nonunion cases, to permit primary bone healing, because no callus is formed during scaphoid healing.

When possible, screw fixation is the preferred technique. However, screws may risk fracturing the bone flap and should be carefully considered. For proximal pole nonunions, if only a cortical shell of bone remains after evacuation of the necrotic bone, the screw threads will not have sufficient purchase in the tenuous shell. In these situations, K-wire fixation is prudent. Symptomatic clicking with wrist flexion can occur with plate fixation after volar VBF surgery requiring subsequent plate removal once union has been achieved.[10]

Volar VBFs are harvested through a volar approach to the wrist. Occasionally, a small dorsal incision may be needed for antegrade screw placement for small proximal pole fractures. A dorsal percutaneous approach can also be used.

VOLAR VASCULARIZED BONE FLAPS

This article describes 4 volar VBFs.

Volar Carpal Artery Vascularized Bone Flap

The volar (or palmar) carpal artery VBF is elevated from the volar-ulnar distal radius epiphysis based on the radial branch of the volar carpal artery and its accompanying 2 vena comitantes.[11] The volar carpal arch arises from the radial and ulnar vessels and runs along the distal edge of the pronator quadratus (**Fig. 1**).[12] The anatomy of the arch is consistent with 3 branches (radial, ulnar, and third interosseous) converging volarly at the distal radioulnar joint (DRUJ). The volar carpal artery VBF is elevated on the dominant branch, and the bone harvest site is designed accordingly for the maximal arc of rotation into the scaphoid defect (**Fig. 2**):

- In 98% of cases, the radial branch is dominant. It travels as an arch from radial to ulnar over the epiphysis of the distal radius 0.5 to 1.5 cm proximal to the radiocarpal joint. When the radial branch is dominant, the bone flap is harvested from the volar-ulnar aspect of the radius.
- In 2% of cases, the ulnar branch is dominant. The flap is elevated from the volar-radial distal radius.

For harvest, a hockey stick incision is used starting with a longitudinal incision over the flexor carpi radialis (FCR) and then angling radially at the volar wrist crease to provide exposure distally over the scaphoid. The FCR and radial artery are mobilized radially and the flexor tendons and median nerve are retracted ulnarly. Deep, the pronator quadratus is exposed and the volar carpal arch is identified at its distal margin, 1 cm proximal to the DRUJ.

The radioscaphocapitate (RSC) ligament is incised and the scaphoid nonunion is identified. Step-cut Z-lengthening of the RSC can facilitate later closure of the volar capsule without compressing the VBF pedicle. The nonunion site is debrided to healthy bleeding bone proximal and distally. K-wire joysticks are used in the proximal and distal scaphoid to facilitate manipulation and reduction.

The VBF dimensions are marked based on the scaphoid defect. The proposed flap location is confirmed with fluoroscopy to avoid injury to the articular cartilage of the radiocarpal joint or DRUJ. The volar cortex of the distal radius flap is measured and cut using an oscillating saw. The flap is levered out of the distal radius using osteotomes. The pedicle is elevated subperiosteally.[13] The tourniquet can be deflated to confirm that the flap is bleeding and arterial pulsations are present within the pedicle. Additional distal radius

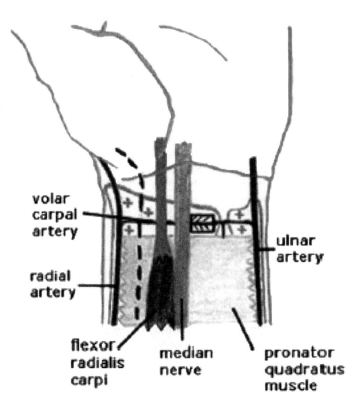

volar carpal artery

radial artery

ulnar artery

flexor radialis carpi

median nerve

pronator quadratus muscle

Fig. 1. The volar carpal arch is located approximately 1 cm proximal to the radiocarpal joint, just distal to the pronator quadratus. It is formed by anastomosing branches of the radial and ulnar arteries. (*Adapted from* Mouilhade F, Auquit-Auckbur I, Duparc F, et al. Anatomical comparative study of two vascularized bone grafts for the wrist. Surg Radiol Anat 2007; 29: 16; with permission.)

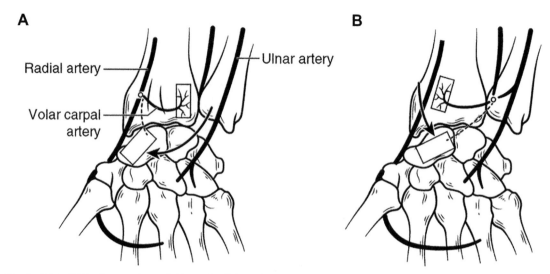

Fig. 2. (*A*) In 98% of cases, the radial branch of the volar carpal artery is dominant and the volar carpal artery VBF is harvested from the volar-ulnar distal radius. (*B*) In 2% of cases, the ulnar branch of the volar carpal artery is dominant and the flap is harvested from the volar-radial distal radius to permit the widest arc of rotation to the scaphoid. (*Adapted from* Kuhlmann JN, Mimoun M, Boabighi A, et al. Vascularized bone graft pedicled on the volar carpal artery for non-union of the scaphoid. J Hand Surg Br 1987;12(2):206; with permission.)

bone can be harvested as cancellous nonvascularized bone graft for packing into the fracture site.

The VBF is passed under the FCR and into the scaphoid defect. Once dissected back to its origin, the elevated pedicle permits the VBF to reach the distal pole of the scaphoid without tension. Mobilization of the radial artery can facilitate distal flap placement. Flap fixation is performed. Fluoroscopy is used to confirm flap placement, adequacy of the internal fixation, restoration of scaphoid anatomy, and correction of any dorsal intercalated segment instability (DISI) deformity. Repair of the RSC, closure of the volar wrist capsule and skin, and splinting is then completed.

A recent study of 9 patients who underwent volar carpal artery VBF and volar plating for scaphoid nonunion with an 11- to 19-month follow-up revealed bone union in 8/9 patients (defined as 50% bone bridging on CT), patient satisfaction in 8/9 patients, 75% grip strength compared with contralateral (improved from the preoperative values), and 60° of wrist flexion and 64° of wrist extension postoperatively (similar to the preoperative values).[10]

Pronator Quadratus Vascularized Bone Flap

The pronator quadratus VBF is elevated from the volar radial styloid with its vascularity based primarily on the insertion of the pronator quadratus. The pronator quadratus VBF is reliable and is commonly used to treat cases of scaphoid

nonunion (**Fig. 3**). The flap's blood supply is provided by the distal transverse strip of pronator quadratus harvested with the flap and from the anterior interosseous artery (AIA) (**Fig. 4**).[14] The AIA provides the dominant blood supply to the pronator quadratus with a consistent branch entering the muscle 2 cm distal to the muscle's proximal edge.[15] The vessel then enters the periosteum over the volar radial styloid and continues into the radius. The pronator quadratus also receives blood supply from anastomoses with the radial and ulnar arteries and rarely from the branches of the posterior interosseous artery.[16] Venous outflow occurs through the vena comitantes into the deep veins of the forearm.[16] A full-thickness strip of pronator quadratus (typically 2 cm thick) should be elevated with a width of at least 2 cm at its insertion into the flap and 4 cm at its proximal ulnar base.[14,17]

The pronator quadratus VBF can reach the distal ulna and the proximal and distal carpal bones.[18] Ligation of vessels entering the pronator quadratus from the radial artery permits increased mobilization of the pronator quadratus pedicle. Subperiosteal elevation of the muscle from the ulna, removal of the superficial pronator quadratus fascia, a 1 cm stretch of the pronator quadratus pedicle, and wrist flexion and forearm pronation can also be used to increase the VBF's arc of rotation. Creation of a shallow groove in the volar distal radius can create a trough for the pedicle for increased reach of the flap distally.[14]

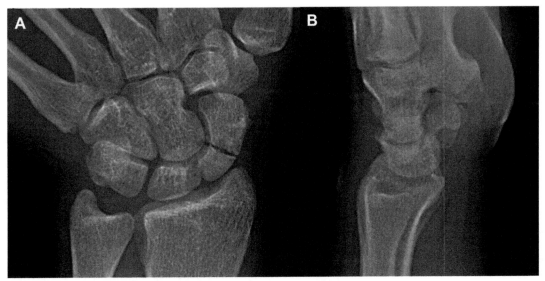

Fig. 3. (*A*) Scaphoid (ulnar deviation) and (*B*) lateral view radiographs of the wrist reveal a 6-month-old scaphoid waist fracture nonunion. Further MRI, not shown here, demonstrated avascular necrosis of the proximal pole and a humpback deformity of the scaphoid in this 22-year-old collegiate football player.

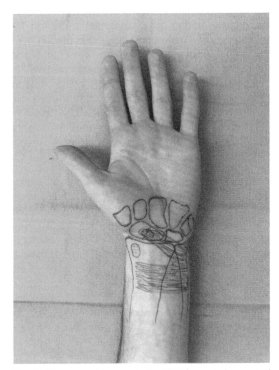

Fig. 4. The pronator quadratus VBF bone is harvested from the volar radial styloid and can be rotated distally to revascularize a scaphoid nonunion. The distal pronator quadratus provides vascularity to the flap. (*Courtesy of* You Jeong Kim, BS, Ann Arbor, Michigan.)

A hockey stick incision is used, similar to the volar carpal artery VBF for harvest (**Fig. 5**). The scaphoid is exposed and the nonunion site is prepared for grafting (**Fig. 6**). The flap size required is measured. The bone for harvest is marked over the volar radial styloid, volar to the abductor pollicis longus (**Fig. 7**).[19] The bone flap is elevated using an oscillating saw and osteotomes to lever it out of the distal radius (**Fig. 8**). The distal pronator quadratus is elevated transversely, with the pedicle flap cuts made in the direction of the oblique fibers of the muscle (from proximal-ulnar to distal-radial). The AIA can often be visualized on the undersurface of the pronator quadratus and is preserved during VBF elevation. After VBF elevation, nonvascularized cancellous bone can be harvested from the volar distal radius using a curette. The VBF is inset, its position is checked under fluoroscopy, and then fixation is performed (**Fig. 9**).

One of the disadvantages of the pronator quadratus VBF is that its muscular leash can be short, limiting distal rotation of the VBF, even when the pronator quadratus is released from the ulna.[20] An advantage is that a more robust pedicle is harvested compared with the volar carpal artery VBF, which has relatively fine vessels and no muscle for protection.

A study of 27 patients with a scaphoid nonunion treated with a pronator quadratus VBF and a headless compression screw demonstrated union in all patients at a mean of 11.5 weeks postoperatively.[8] Radiographic carpal alignment improved, grip

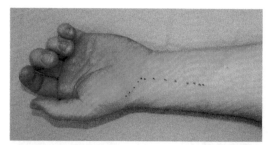

Fig. 5. A hockey stick incision is used for harvest of the pronator quadratus pedicled VBF and placement into the scaphoid nonunion site volarly.

strength compared with contralateral was 82% to 91%, and wrist range of motion compared with contralateral was 84% for flexion and 81% for extension postoperatively.

Volar Distal Ulna Vascularized Bone Flap

The distal ulna VBF is based on retrograde flow through the ulnar artery.[21] Bone from the ulnar aspect of the distal third of the ulna is harvested, up to 3 cm in length and one-third of the diameter of the diaphysis width, with the overlying periosteum. The ulnar artery gives off a reliable branch to the distal third of the ulna, traversing through the flexor carpi ulnaris (FCU). The ulnar artery is harvested as the pedicle with a cuff of FCU muscle around the perforator entering the VBF. After harvest, ulnar artery reconstruction with a vein graft is recommended. A patent palmar arch with a normal Allen test must be present preoperatively and reassessed intraoperatively before ulnar artery division to avoid ischemia of the hand. Doppler ultrasound and/or computed tomographic (CT)

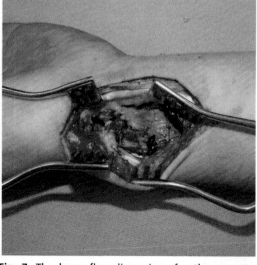

Fig. 7. The bone flap dimensions for the pronator quadratus VBF are marked over the volar radial styloid.

angiography should be obtained in patients who have had multiple previous radial wrist surgeries to confirm the patency of the radial artery before surgery.

Two longitudinal incisions are used. The first is designed over the volar-ulnar distal forearm for flap elevation. The second incision is placed over the volar-radial wrist for flap inset into the scaphoid (**Fig. 10**). The vascular pedicle is dissected to Guyon canal, which is the rotation point for the VBF. The ulnar nerve must be protected.

Guimberteau and Panconi treated 8 patients with this technique. All patients achieved bone

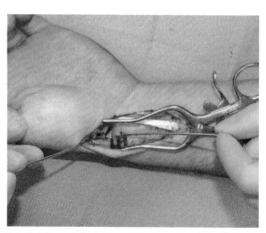

Fig. 6. The scaphoid nonunion site is identified and debrided back to bleeding bone. K-wire joysticks are placed in the proximal and distal scaphoid to assist with manipulation and reduction.

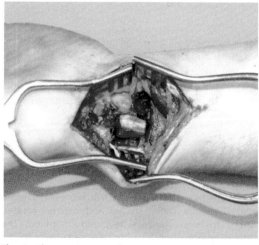

Fig. 8. The corticocancellous pronator quadratus VBF is elevated using osteotomes.

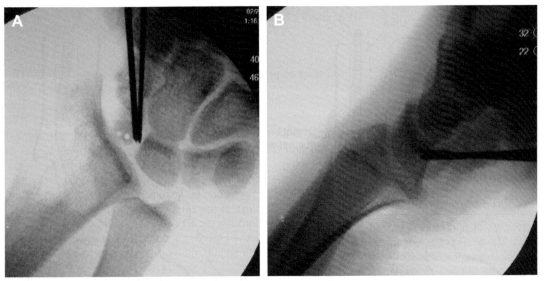

Fig. 9. (A) Posteroanterior (PA) and (B) lateral fluoroscopic images reveal placement of the VBF and K-wire fixation at the scaphoid waist nonunion site with restoration of scaphoid height and correction of the humpback deformity.

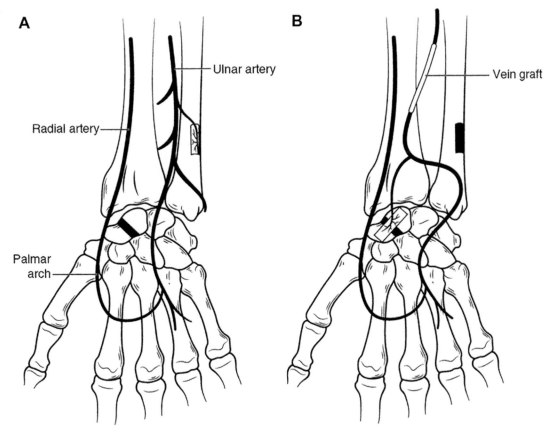

Fig. 10. (A) The distal ulna VBF is harvested from the ulnar aspect of the distal third of the ulna based on the ulnar artery and then (B) rotated into the scaphoid. (B) A vein graft is used to reconstruct the ulnar artery. (*Adapted from* Guimberteau JC, Panconi B. Recalcitrant non-union of the scaphoid treated with a vascularized bone graft based on the ulnar artery. J Bone Joint Surg Am 1990;72(1):88-97; with permission.)

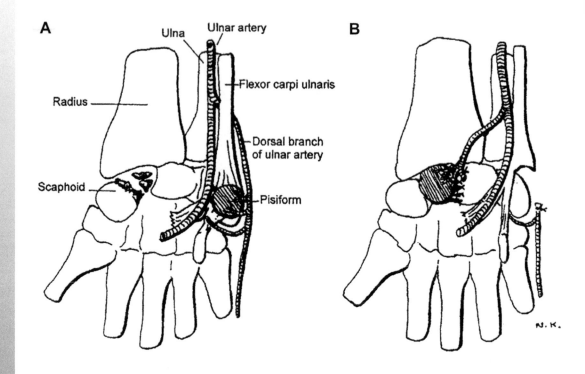

Fig. 11. (A) The pisiform is dissected away from the FCU with its vascularity maintained by the dorsal branch of the ulnar artery. (B) Vessels entering the radial aspect of the pisiform and the dorsal carpal branch of the ulnar artery are divided to permit adequate mobility for placement of the VBF into the volar scaphoid. (*Adapted from* Kuhlmann JN, Kron C, Boabighi A, et al. Vascularised pisiform bone graft. Indications, technique and long-term results. Acta Orthop Belg 2003;69(4):312; with permission.)

union (average 4.6 months post-op) and resumed their previous occupational and athletic activities.[21] Harvesting the ulnar artery as the VBF pedicle, the risk of injury to the ulnar nerve, and the palpable defect that results in the ulnar aspect of the ulna are disadvantages of this donor site. The distal ulna volar VBF is included in this article for completeness but is not a first-line option for treatment of scaphoid nonunions due to the morbidity of the ulnar artery harvest.

Pisiform Vascularized Bone Flap

The vascularized pisiform bone flap is based on the dorsal branch of the ulnar artery. The pedicle is typically over 4 cm long allowing the flap to reach the scaphoid and the lunate. The pisiform VBF can be used to replace the proximal pole of the scaphoid, because it approximates the shape of the proximal pole well and is covered by articular cartilage.[22] When used as an intercalary bone flap, due to the small size of the pisiform VBF, the scaphoid will typically lose some height.

An incision is made longitudinally over the volar distal forearm and wrist, just radial to the FCU

tendon. The pisiform is freed from the FCU and the pisohamate ligament is divided. The vessels entering the radial side of the pisiform are divided and the ulnar sided vessels are preserved. The pisotriquetral capsule is opened and harvested with the pisiform VBF. The dorsal branch of the ulnar artery is dissected and divided distal to the pisiform to permit radial movement of the VBF (**Fig. 11**). The VBF is dissected away from the ulnar nerve and passed under the FCU.

The transverse carpal ligament is opened. The flexor tendons and median nerve are retracted radially and the VBF is passed deep to reach the scaphoid after opening the volar-radial wrist capsule. The pisotriquetral capsule is sutured to the remnants of the scapholunate ligament on the lunate when the VBF is used to replace the proximal pole of the scaphoid.

In their article, Kuhlmann and colleagues[22] reported on 14 patients who had vascularized pisiform grafting (12 men, 2 women; 7 with AVN of the scaphoid, and 7 with Kienbock disease). All patients had a minimum of 1 year follow-up; 8 patients had more than 5-year follow-up. K-wire fixation was used. For the patients with scaphoid

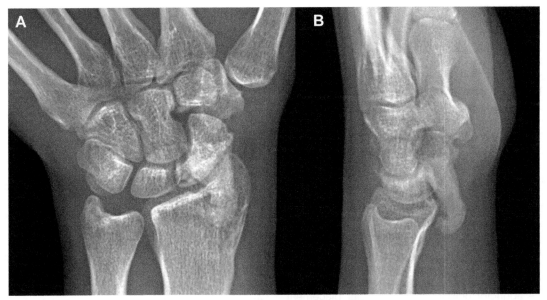

Fig. 12. (*A*) PA and (*B*) lateral X rays done 6 months postoperatively reveal complete bony union after a pronator quadratus VBF for scaphoid nonunion. Asymptomatic calcification of the pronator quadratus muscle can be observed radiographically.

reconstruction, bone healing occurred in all, wrist flexion and extension was 10° to 30° less and grip strength was 10% to 20% less than the contralateral side, and pain resolved in 6/7 patients (1 failure occurred in a patient in whom the VBF was not properly placed; it did not articulate with the scaphoid fossa of the radius, and the patient went on to a total wrist fusion). Two out of seven patients had postoperative hyperesthesia and dysesthesia in the ulnar nerve distribution. At 5- to 12-year follow-up, no further pain was reported and the clinical and radiographic results were unchanged from the 1-year postoperative results.

The vascularized pisiform VBF is the only pedicled VBF covered by articular cartilage. If the entire proximal pole of the scaphoid requires replacement, it is the most suitable regional choice. A medial femoral trochlear free flap is another option but requires a distant donor site.

POSTOPERATIVE CARE

Immobilization is used until clinical and radiographic signs of healing are noted. Generally below-elbow casting is used for 6 weeks followed by 4 weeks of full-time splint use. Longer periods of immobilization are often needed for long-standing nonunions (3–4 months). Posteroanterior and lateral X rays are performed routinely in the postoperative period (**Fig. 12**). Approximately 3 months postoperatively, CT imaging is performed to confirm more than 50% trabecular

bone bridging before weaning patients out of their splints and return to full activities. Hand therapy is prescribed to guide range of motion and strengthening exercises (**Fig. 13**).

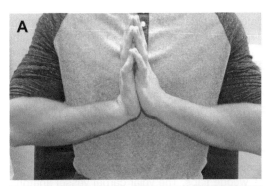

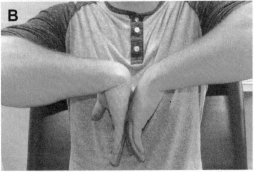

Fig. 13. Eight months after scaphoid nonunion treatment with a pronator quadratus VBF, the patient had regained functional wrist extension (*A*) and (*B*) flexion and had been able to return to football without pain.

DISCUSSION

The volar carpal arch and pronator quadratus VBFs are the most commonly used volar VBFs for scaphoid nonunion. They provide corticocancellous flaps with minimal donor site morbidity. The ulnar nerve is at risk of injury with the distal ulna and pisiform VBFs. The pisiform VBF is an option for replacement of the proximal pole of the scaphoid but is often too small for intercalary scaphoid defects. The ulnar VBF requires harvest of the ulnar artery, which can lead to hand ischemia.

Dorsal carpal VBFs are used more commonly than volar VBFs.[23] The most commonly used dorsal VBFs are the 1,2 and 2,3 intercompartmental supraretinacular arteries (ICSRA) and the 4 + 5 extracompartmental artery flaps. The 1,2 ICSRA bone flap can be harvested from a radial incision over the distal wrist and passed radially under the abductor pollicis longus for volar placement into a scaphoid nonunion site.[24]

A dorsal VBF can also be harvested from the dorsal base of the index finger metacarpal based on the second dorsal metacarpal artery.[25] If this vessel is damaged during harvest, the third dorsal metacarpal artery can be used as an alternative pedicle. At the level of the base of the metacarpals, the second metacarpal artery is over 1 mm in diameter. For patients with a DISI deformity, volar inset of this VBF is recommended; in those without malalignment of the carpus, a dorsal approach is used. The flap is harvested dorsally and then can be passed under the abductor pollicis longus and extensor pollicis brevis tendons for insertion into the volar scaphoid.

Advantages of volar flaps include the ability to approach the scaphoid volarly facilitating correction of humpback deformity and restoration of scaphoid height.[24] The flaps are gently impacted as wedge flaps. The volar carpal vessel anatomy is more consistent than the dorsal carpal vessels.[26] Disadvantages of volar VBFs include the risk of carpal instability and ulnar translation of the carpus due to ligamentous disruption from a volar approach. Injuries to the median nerve (palmar cutaneous branch or proper nerve), radial artery, or ulnar artery or nerve can occur. The dorsal approach to the scaphoid and use of a dorsal VBF provide an improved ability to visualize the proximal pole of the scaphoid and the dorsal scapholunate ligament but have a higher risk of damaging the dorsal scaphoid branches of the radial artery entering the dorsal ridge of the scaphoid that supply the proximal 70% to 80% of the scaphoid.[27]

The thick volar cortical bone harvested with the volar carpal artery and pronator quadratus VBFs provides robust structural support for the volar scaphoid after correction of a humpback deformity. The dorsal cortex of the radius is thinner and the 1,2 ICSRA can be insufficient for restoring scaphoid height. The cancellous bone of the volar radius is more compacted and adherent to the overlying volar cortical bone compared with the dorsal cancellous bone of the distal radius permitting easier inset of a volar VBF compared with a dorsal VBF with less risk of damage to the flap during impaction into a scaphoid nonunion defect and fixation.

The volar carpal artery VBF has a longer pedicle than the dorsal 1,2 ICSRA VBF.[26] Both flaps can reach the scaphoid. The volar carpal artery VBF reaches the lunate in all cases, whereas the 1,2 ICSRA can reach in 80% of cases.[26] For scapholunate fusions requiring augmentation with a VBF, the volar carpal artery flap can be used, and the 1,2 ICSRA will not reach. The 1,2 ICSRA will reach the lunotriquetral joint, scaphotrapezial joint, and trapezium.

SUMMARY

Multiple options exist, from both the volar and dorsal distal radius, for pedicled VBF reconstruction for scaphoid nonunion. Choice of VBF depends primarily on the scaphoid defect (location of the nonunion, presence of AVN and/or humpback deformity, history of previous surgery, and possible resultant pedicle damage). The 4 volar VBFs described in this article provide versatile options for scaphoid reconstruction.

REFERENCES

1. Kara T, Gunal I. Preiser's disease treated by pronator quadratus pedicled bone graft. J Plast Surg Hand Surg 2014;48(6):455–6.
2. Shin AY, Bishop AT. Vascularized bone grafts for scaphoid nonunions and kienböck's disease. Orthop Clin North Am 2001;32(2):263–77, viii.
3. Munk B, Larsen CF. Bone grafting the scaphoid nonunion: a systematic review of 147 publications including 5,246 cases of scaphoid nonunion. Acta Orthop Scand 2004;75(5):618–29.
4. Higgins JP, Burger HK. Proximal scaphoid arthroplasty using the medial femoral trochlea flap. J Wrist Surg 2013;2(3):228–33.
5. Bürger HK, Windhofer C, Gaggl AJ, et al. Vascularized medial femoral trochlea osteocartilaginous flap reconstruction of proximal pole scaphoid nonunions. J Hand Surg Am 2013; 38(4):690–700.

6. Harpf C, Gabl M, Reinhart C, et al. Small free vascularized iliac crest bone grafts in reconstruction of the scaphoid bone: a retrospective study in 60 cases. Plast Reconstr Surg 2001;108(3):664–74.

7. Lanzetta M. Scaphoid reconstruction by a free vascularized osteochondral graft from the rib: a case report. Microsurgery 2009;29(5):420–4.

8. Lee SK, Park JS, Choy WS. Scaphoid fracture nonunion treated with pronator quadratus pedicled vascularized bone graft and headless compression screw. Ann Plast Surg 2015;74(6):665–71.

9. Dodds SD, Patterson JT, Halim A. Volar plate fixation of recalcitrant scaphoid nonunions with volar carpal artery vascularized bone graft. Tech Hand Up Extrem Surg 2014;18(1):2–7.

10. Dodds SD, Halim A. Scaphoid plate fixation and volar carpal artery vascularized bone graft for recalcitrant scaphoid nonunions. J Hand Surg Am 2016; 41(7):e191–8.

11. Kuhlmann JN, Mimoun M, Boabighi A, et al. Vascularized bone graft pedicled on the volar carpal artery for non-union of the scaphoid. J Hand Surg Br 1987; 12(2):203–10.

12. Mathoulin C, Haerle M. Vascularized bone graft from the palmar carpal artery for treatment of scaphoid nonunion. J Hand Surg Br 1998;23(3):318–23.

13. Dailiana ZH, Malizos KN, Zachos V, et al. Vascularized bone grafts from the palmar radius for the treatment of waist nonunions of the scaphoid. J Hand Surg Am 2006;31(3):397–404.

14. Lee JC, Lim J, Chacha PB. The anatomical basis of the vascularized pronator quadratus pedicled bone graft. J Hand Surg Br 1997;22(5):644–6.

15. Rath S, Hung LK, Leung PC. Vascular anatomy of the pronator quadratus muscle-bone flap: a justification for its use with a distally based blood supply. J Hand Surg Am 1990;15(4):630–6.

16. Papp C, Maurer H, Ausserlechner M, et al. Reconstruction of pseudarthrosis of the scaphoid bone utilizing an osteomuscular pronator quadratus transposition flap. Eur J Plast Surg 1993;16(6):257–62.

17. Noaman HH, Shiha AE, Ibrahim AK. Functional outcomes of nonunion scaphoid fracture treated by pronator quadratus pedicled bone graft. Ann Plast Surg 2011;66(1):47–52.

18. Leung PC, Hung LK. Use of pronator quadratus bone flap in bony reconstruction around the wrist. J Hand Surg Am 1990;15(4):637–40.

19. Kawai H, Yamamoto K. Pronator quadratus pedicled bone graft for old scaphoid fractures. J Bone Joint Surg Br 1988;70(5):829–31.

20. Tang P, Fischer CR. A new volar vascularization technique using the superficial palmar branch of the radial artery for the collapsed scaphoid nonunion. Tech Hand Up Extrem Surg 2010;14(3): 160–72.

21. Guimberteau JC, Panconi B. Recalcitrant non-union of the scaphoid treated with a vascularized bone graft based on the ulnar artery. J Bone Joint Surg Am 1990;72(1):88–97.

22. Kuhlmann JN, Kron C, Boabighi A, et al. Vascularised pisiform bone graft. Indications, technique and long-term results. Acta Orthop Belg 2003; 69(4):311–6.

23. Rizzo M, Moran SL. Vascularized bone grafts and their applications in the treatment of carpal pathology. Semin Plast Surg 2008;22(3):213–27.

24. Trumble T, Nyland W. Scaphoid nonunions. Pitfalls and pearls. Hand Clin 2001;17(4):611–24.

25. Sawaizumi T, Nanno M, Nanbu A, et al. Vascularised bone graft from the base of the second metacarpal for refractory nonunion of the scaphoid. J Bone Joint Surg Br 2004;86(7):1007–12.

26. Mouilhade F, Auquit-Auckbur I, Duparc F, et al. Anatomical comparative study of two vascularized bone grafts for the wrist. Surg Radiol Anat 2007; 29(1):15–20.

27. Gelberman RH, Menon J. The vascularity of the scaphoid bone. J Hand Surg Am 1980;5(5):508–13.

Managing the Athlete with a Scaphoid Fracture

Edward W. Jernigan, MD, Kyle W. Morse, MD*, Michelle G. Carlson, MD

KEYWORDS

- Scaphoid fracture • Athlete • Wrist injuries • Scaphoid surgery • Wrist surgery
- Scaphoid fracture healing

KEY POINTS

- Most minimally displaced scaphoid fractures and all displaced scaphoid fractures in elite athletes are treated with early fixation to maximally expedite the return to full function.
- Preoperative computed tomographic (CT) scans are recommended in all scaphoid fractures to facilitate a complete understanding of fracture anatomy to allow for optimal screw placement.
- Screw placement is important to maximize healing capacity of the fracture to allow for return to sport.
- Postoperative CT scans can be helpful to evaluate the extent of healing and may allow patients to return to play sooner.
- Decisions related to return to play in elite athletes with scaphoid fractures can be difficult and must be individualized to meet the needs of each patient.

INTRODUCTION

Upper extremity fractures are common in elite athletes, and the scaphoid is the most commonly injured carpal bone. Prompt diagnosis of scaphoid fractures in elite athletes is of paramount importance to minimize time away from sport and any complications that can arise from a delay in diagnosis. The goal in treatment of scaphoid fractures in the elite athlete is to expedite healing so that the athlete may return to sport. Surgical treatment of scaphoid fractures requires careful evaluation of each specific fracture pattern, and treatment must be individualized for each athlete. Decision regarding return to play (RTP) is one of the most challenging decisions that surgeons make, with possible ethical, financial, and legal decision implications.

ESTABLISHING THE DIAGNOSIS (X RAY VS COMPUTED TOMOGRAPHIC VS MRI)

Plain radiographs should be obtained in all patients with clinical suspicion of a scaphoid fracture. In addition to the standard AP, lateral, and oblique views, Cooney and colleagues[1] recommend consideration of radioulnar deviation stress views or traction oblique views. With literature demonstrating the low sensitivity of X rays and the detection of scaphoid fractures, and some studies noting sensitivity as low as 70% in adults and 54% in kids, MRI can be helpful in definitively ruling in or out a minimally displaced scaphoid fracture.[2,3] CT and MRI have been shown to have comparable diagnostic characteristics, but the decision on whether MRI or CT scan should be obtained to confirm a radiographic occult scaphoid fracture is controversial.[4,5] There is increasing interest in using cone beam CT, a technique which has been widely implemented in dental as well as head and neck surgery.[6,7] Lower radiation levels than regular CT scan, faster study time relative to MRI, and improved sensitivity relative to plain radiographs may lead to increased utilization of this modality in the years to come; however further research is needed before widespread utilization. Early cross-

The authors have no commercial or financial conflicts of interest or funding sources to disclose.
Division of Hand and Upper Extremity Surgery, Hospital for Special Surgery, 523 East 72nd Street, FL 4, New York, NY 10021, USA
* Corresponding author.
E-mail address: morsek@HSS.EDU

Hand Clin 35 (2019) 365–371
https://doi.org/10.1016/j.hcl.2019.03.011

sectional imaging has been shown to decrease morbidity for patients and overall costs to society and health care systems.[8–10] In the case of a professional athlete with a possible scaphoid fracture, delay in the diagnosis or treatment can lead to large sums of lost wages, and thus strong consideration should be given for early cross-sectional imaging in any athlete with radial-sided wrist pain after an injury in the setting of negative radiographs.

CHARACTERIZATION OF THE FRACTURE PATTERN

Once the diagnosis of a scaphoid fracture has been established, an understanding of fracture morphology can assist the surgeon in establishing an appropriate operative plan, including the best approach, method of fixation, and screw trajectory. CT scan has been shown to improve the reliability of detecting displacement of scaphoid fractures[11,12] (**Fig. 1**). In a recent study of 124 scaphoid fractures, CT scans demonstrated an average angle between the scaphoid longitudinal axis and the fracture to be 53°.[13] Another study of 34 patients comparing diagnosing scaphoid fractures with CT scan reformatted along the axis of the scaphoid versus anatomic axis of the wrist showed improved performance characteristics; however, this did not reach statistical significance.[14] Given the importance in understanding the pattern of the specific fracture, including the obliquity of the fracture line as well as any comminution, the authors recommend obtaining CT scans as part of the workup for any athlete with a scaphoid fracture.

SCAPHOID STRESS FRACTURES

There are several reports of scaphoid stress fractures in the young athlete, both before and after skeletal maturity. These reports describe athletes in a variety of sports, including gymnastics, diving, racket sports, goalkeeping, and shot-putting.[15–19] The mechanism is thought to be related to repetitive hyperextension activities.[15,17] Treatment for stress fractures of the scaphoid in athletes has ranged from conservative management to screw internal fixation. Scaphoid stress fractures, although uncommon, should be on the differential in athletes, especially those who participate in activities requiring repetitive extremes of motion and force applied across of the wrist.

DECISION FOR SURGERY

With the exception of scaphoid tubercle fractures that can generally be treated successfully with nonoperative management, scaphoid fractures in athletes are most often treated surgically to allow expedited return to high-level activity. Even in nondisplaced fractures, surgical treatment results in better functional outcomes, faster return to work, and faster time to union.[20,21] Delayed treatment for scaphoid fractures has been associated with worse outcomes and longer time to union.[22] There is histologic evidence that the healing capacity of the distal portion of the scaphoid decreases with increasing time from injury.[23] In addition, displaced fractures have a higher risk of nonunion than nondisplaced fractures.[24] Therefore, the authors usually do not recommend immobilization to allow for completion of the season even in

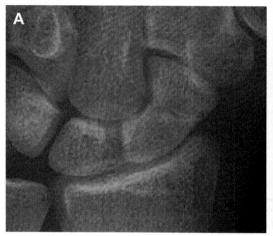
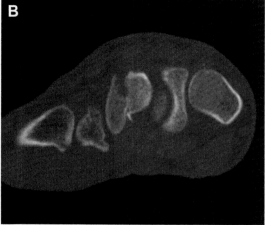

Fig. 1. The use of CT is necessary to describe scaphoid fracture displacement. (*A*) The image demonstrates what seems to be a nondisplaced scaphoid fracture. (*B*) After a CT scan was performed, there is significant displacement of the fracture noted. ([*B*] *From* Gilley E, Puri SK, Hearns KA, et al. Importance of computed tomography in determining displacement in scaphoid fractures. J Wrist Surg 2018;7(1):41; with permission.)

situations where cast immobilization may be allowed, because both the delay in surgical treatment as well as the risk of displacement may put the patient at higher risk for poor outcome.

SURGICAL CONSIDERATIONS

Scaphoid fractures can be approached dorsally or volarly. The primary determinant of approach is morphology of the fracture. The authors favor a dorsal approach for fractures of the proximal pole or scaphoid waist and a volar approach for more distal fractures or in the setting of comminution requiring bone graft or a humpback deformity (**Fig. 2**). There are a variety of commercially available headless screws that allow for placement of a buried screw within the scaphoid, imparting compression across fracture through the variable pitch of the threads. In the setting of extreme comminution, or treatment of subacute scaphoid fractures where there has been resorption of the bone, there has been increasing interest in using either 2 headless compression screws or a plate to increase rotational stability.[25] There have been several biomechanical data suggesting a benefit with 2 screws or a plate compared with a single screw; however there are limited clinical data comparing these methods.[25–29] Further research is indicated to determine whether these constructs increase overall healing rates or decrease time to union relative to more conventional single screw fixation. In most of the cases, the senior author uses a single headless compression screw with

or without distal radius bone graft to achieve fixation.

There is debate in the literature regarding whether headless compression screws should be placed centrally in the scaphoid or perpendicular to the fracture.[30–33] Biomechanical studies have demonstrated similar stiffness and load to failure with screws perpendicular to the fracture versus those placed centrally, despite the screw perpendicular to the fracture being shorter than a central screw.[31,32] Placement of a screw perpendicular to the fracture has been shown to result in higher compressive loads and also increase the amount of surface area between the fragments[33,34] (**Fig. 3**). Therefore, the authors recommend placement of the headless compression screw perpendicular to the fracture in waist fractures. In proximal pole fractures the proximal fragment may be too small to allow for this, and primary concern should be screw purchase of the proximal pole. Studies evaluating bone density in the scaphoid have demonstrated that the subchondral 2 mm shell of the bone has the greatest density, and there is a significant drop-off in bone density away from this 2 mm shell. Therefore, subchondral placement of the headless compression screws may be helpful for increasing strength of fixation.[35]

POSTOPERATIVE COMPUTED TOMOGRAPHIC SCAN TO ASSESS HEALING

Given concerns regarding the reliability of using plain radiographs to evaluate for scaphoid

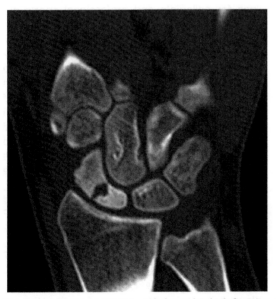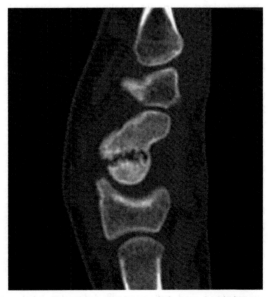

Fig. 2. Scaphoid nonunion with humpback deformity. Coronal and sagittal CT views of the scaphoid demonstrating the dorsal humpback deformity. The distal fragment can be seen in a flexed posture while the proximal fragment is extended. To correct this deformity, the authors recommend a volar approach to the scaphoid.

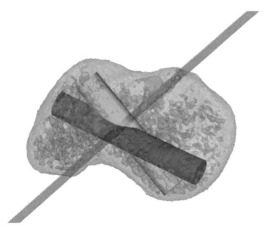

Fig. 3. Three-dimensional reconstruction of a middle-third scaphoid fracture with multiple screw trajectories. The reconstruction demonstrates a fracture plane through the scaphoid waist (*horizontal red line*), perpendicular screw placement (*green cylinder*), and central pole to pole placement (*red cylinder*). (*From* Swanstrom MM, Morse KW, Lipman JD, et al. Effect of screw perpendicularity on compression in scaphoid waist fractures. J Wrist Surg 2017;6(3):179; with permission.)

fracture healing, the use of CT scan to assess postoperative healing has gained popularity.[36,37] Determining healing of a scaphoid fracture can be challenging regardless of the imaging modality, and much of the current literature on the rate of bridging callus formation across scaphoid fractures has focused on nonoperatively managed fractures. Grewal and colleagues[37] characterized scaphoid healing in a cohort of 66 patients treated nonoperatively. The first CT scan in these patients was obtained between 12 and 18 weeks after injury. In a subset of 22 patients with partial union noted on their 12 to 18 week CT scan, 10 patients had 75% to 99% union, 7 had 50% to 74% union, and 5 had 25% to 49% union. In their series, all patients with partial union noted at the 12 to 18 week postinjury CT scan went on to union, including those with only 25% to 50% bridging bone. In a cohort of 59 patients treated nonoperatively, Geoghegan and colleagues[38] demonstrated 43 of 59 patients with scaphoid waste fractures treated nonoperatively to be united with greater than 50% bridging across the fracture on a 4-week postinjury CT scan. The literature may benefit from further study evaluating progression of partial unions to full union in operatively treated fractures. More recent literature from Clementson and colleagues[39] defined a healed fracture as one that demonstrated a continuous trabecular pattern over more than 50% of the

cross-sectional area of the fracture, and reported in a series of 15 patients treated operatively a union rate of 80% at 6 weeks and 93% at 10 weeks. In a series of patients with proximal pole fractures, Grewal and colleagues[40] using a similar definition report a time to union at mean 14 weeks in operatively treated patients. Given much of the literature that has characterized rates of bridging callus across the fracture in nonoperatively treated fractures, further research is indicated to explore rate of bridging callus across the fracture after operative treatment.[41]

RETURN TO COMPETITION

RTP decisions are one of the most challenging decisions facing the surgeon treating elite athletes and must be determined on an individual basis. Patient-specific characteristics, including fracture morphology, sport, position, as well as professional organization formal guidelines, should be taken into account when determining when an elite athlete may RTP. Decisions regarding RTP can also be associated with ethical dilemmas of the treating physician related to a sense of shared responsibility to athletes, team management, and the respective sport's governing body.[42] The morphology of the fracture also plays a role in the RTP determination. Minimally displaced scaphoid waist fractures tend to heal quickly and allow for expeditious RTP; however, proximal or more displaced fractures may take longer to heal and thus delay RTP. Protective play guidelines for collegiate and professional sports are highly variable.[43] For example, a hockey player may wear protective devices under their gloves, whereas this would not be an option for a basketball player.[44,45] Within football, some positions are better suited for protected play, such as linemen and defensive players, whereas receivers and quarterbacks may not be able to perform with protective splints.[46] A survey of professional team surgeons demonstrated that 51% allowed athletes to return to unprotected play 4 to 6 weeks after open reduction internal fixation (ORIF) of a nondisplaced scaphoid fracture. In the survey, 32% allowed immediate return to protected play. With regard to unprotected play after ORIF of a nondisplaced scaphoid fracture, 24% allowed for RTP at 4 to 6 weeks, 49% at 6 to 12 weeks, and 27% at greater than 12 weeks.[47] In general, once a postoperative CT scan demonstrates bridging of 50% of the fracture site and the player has regained full range of motion, the authors believe return to unprotected play is possible.

ETHICS

Navigating the physician-patient-team relationship can be challenging and it leads to ethical conflict between parties. There is no universally accepted code of sports medicine ethics, leading to further challenges for the physician treating elite athletes.[48] Factors including the physician's employer, the athlete's desire to play with pain and injury with the potential for a poorer long-term outcome, and economic considerations for the patient can lead to unique treatment and disclosure-related issues for any physician treating the elite athlete.[49] One of the complexities of treatment of the elite athlete is the issue of patient confidentiality.[50,51] In a survey of 45 sports medicine physicians, the most commonly mentioned ethical issue in sports medicine was issues related to confidentiality and privacy.[42] The Health Insurance Portability and Accountability Act (HIPPA) of 1996 set forth privacy regulations with the goal of protecting patient health information. Magee and colleagues[52] analyzed the role of HIPPA in the treatment of professional athletes, concluding that information obtained by a team physician may be part of the employment record and thus not considered protected health information (PHI). In comparison, information is considered PHI when a physician is treating an athlete and the physician is not employed by the team or when an examination is performed in a private office; in these cases HIPPA guidelines apply for the protection of the patient.[52]

SUMMARY

Most minimally displaced scaphoid fractures and all displaced scaphoid fractures in elite athletes are treated with early fixation to maximally expedite the return to full function. Preoperative CT scans are recommended in all scaphoid fractures to facilitate a complete understanding of fracture anatomy to allow for optimal screw placement. Screw placement is important to maximize healing capacity of the fracture to allow for return to sport. Postoperative CT scans can be helpful to evaluate the extent of healing and may allow patients to RTP sooner. Decisions related to RTP in elite athletes with scaphoid fractures can be challenging and must be individualized to meet the needs of each patient.

REFERENCES

1. Cooney WP, Dobyns JH, Linscheid RL. Fractures of the scaphoid: a rational approach to management. Clin Orthop Relat Res 1980;149:90–7.

2. Jørgsholm P, Thomsen N, Besjakov J, et al. MRI shows a high incidence of carpal fractures in children with posttraumatic radial-sided wrist tenderness. Acta Orthop 2016;87(5):533–7.

3. Jørgsholm P, Thomsen NOB, Besjakov J, et al. The benefit of magnetic resonance imaging for patients with posttraumatic radial wrist tenderness. J Hand Surg Am 2013;38(1):29–33.

4. Mallee W, Doornberg JN, Ring D, et al. Comparison of CT and MRI for diagnosis of suspected scaphoid fractures. J Bone Joint Surg Am 2011; 93(1):20–8.

5. Yin Z-G, Zhang J-B, Kan S-L, et al. Diagnosing suspected scaphoid fractures: a systematic review and meta-analysis. Clin Orthop Relat Res 2010;468(3): 723–34.

6. Edlund R, Skorpil M, Lapidus G, et al. Cone-beam CT in diagnosis of scaphoid fractures. Skeletal Radiol 2016;45(2):197–204.

7. Borel C, Larbi A, Delclaux S, et al. Diagnostic value of cone beam computed tomography (CBCT) in occult scaphoid and wrist fractures. Eur J Radiol 2017;97:59–64.

8. Hansen TB, Petersen RB, Barckman J, et al. Cost-effectiveness of MRI in managing suspected scaphoid fractures. J Hand Surg Eur Vol 2009; 34(5):627–30.

9. Patel NK, Davies N, Mirza Z, et al. Cost and clinical effectiveness of MRI in occult scaphoid fractures: a randomised controlled trial. Emerg Med J 2013; 30(3):202–7.

10. Karl JW, Swart E, Strauch RJ. Diagnosis of occult scaphoid fractures: a cost-effectiveness analysis. J Bone Joint Surg Am 2015;97(22):1860–8.

11. Lozano-Calderón S, Blazar P, Zurakowski D, et al. Diagnosis of scaphoid fracture displacement with radiography and computed tomography. J Bone Joint Surg Am 2006;88(12):2695–703.

12. Gilley E, Puri SK, Hearns KA, et al. Importance of computed tomography in determining displacement in scaphoid fractures. J Wrist Surg 2018;7(1):38–42.

13. Luria S, Schwarcz Y, Wollstein R, et al. 3-dimensional analysis of scaphoid fracture angle morphology. J Hand Surg Am 2015;40(3):508–14.

14. Mallee WH, Doornberg JN, Ring D, et al. Computed tomography for suspected scaphoid fractures: comparison of reformations in the plane of the wrist versus the long axis of the scaphoid. Hand (N Y) 2014;9(1):117–21.

15. Kohyama S, Kanamori A, Tanaka T, et al. Stress fracture of the scaphoid in an elite junior tennis player: a case report and review of the literature. J Med Case Rep 2016;10:8.

16. Mohamed Haflah NH, Mat Nor NF, Abdullah S, et al. Bilateral scaphoid stress fracture in a platform diver presenting with unilateral symptoms. Singapore Med J 2014;55(10):e159–61.

17. Pidemunt G, Torres-Claramunt R, Ginés A, et al. Bilateral stress fracture of the carpal scaphoid:' ' report in a child and review of the literature. Clin J Sport Med 2012;22(6):511–3.

18. Kohring JM, Curtiss HM, Tyser AR. A scaphoid stress fracture in a female collegiate-level shot-putter and review of the literature. Case Rep Orthop 2016;2016:8098657.

19. Nakamoto JC, Saito M, Cunha AP, et al. Scaphoid stress fracture in gymnastics athlete: a case report. Rev Bras Ortop 2009;44(6):533–5.

20. Al-Ajmi TA, Al-Faryan KH, Al-Kanaan NF, et al. A systematic review and meta-analysis of randomized controlled trials comparing surgical versus conservative treatments for acute undisplaced or minimally-displaced scaphoid fractures. Clin Orthop Surg 2018;10(1):64–73.

21. Buijze GA, Doornberg JN, Ham JS, et al. Surgical compared with conservative treatment for acute nondisplaced or minimally displaced scaphoid fractures: a systematic review and meta-analysis of randomized controlled trials. J Bone Joint Surg Am 2010;92(6):1534–44.

22. Wong K, von Schroeder HP. Delays and poor management of scaphoid fractures: factors contributing to nonunion. J Hand Surg Am 2011;36(9):1471–4.

23. Schmidle G, Ebner HL, Klima G, et al. Time-dependent changes in bone healing capacity of scaphoid fractures and non-unions. J Anat 2018;232(6):908–18.

24. Singh HP, Taub N, Dias JJ. Management of displaced fractures of the waist of the scaphoid: meta-analyses of comparative studies. Injury 2012;43(6):933–9.

25. Jurkowitsch J, Dall'Ara E, Quadlbauer S, et al. Rotational stability in screw-fixed scaphoid fractures compared to plate-fixed scaphoid fractures. Arch Orthop Trauma Surg 2016;136(11):1623–8.

26. Quadlbauer S, Beer T, Pezzei C, et al. Stabilization of scaphoid type B2 fractures with one or two headless compression screws. Arch Orthop Trauma Surg 2017;137(11):1587–95.

27. Dodds SD, Williams JB, Seiter M, et al. Lessons learned from volar plate fixation of scaphoid fracture nonunions. J Hand Surg Eur Vol 2018;43(1):57–65.

28. Goodwin JA, Castañeda P, Shelhamer RP, et al. A comparison of plate versus screw fixation for segmental scaphoid fractures: a biomechanical study. Hand (N Y) 2017. https://doi.org/10.1177/1558944717732065.

29. Mandaleson A, Tham SK, Lewis C, et al. Scaphoid fracture fixation in a nonunion model: a biomechanical study comparing 3 types of fixation. J Hand Surg Am 2018;43(3):221–8.

30. Dodds SD, Panjabi MM, Slade JF. Screw fixation of scaphoid fractures: a biomechanical assessment of screw length and screw augmentation. J Hand Surg Am 2006;31(3):405–13.

31. Faucher GK, Golden ML, Sweeney KR, et al. Comparison of screw trajectory on stability of oblique scaphoid fractures: a mechanical study. J Hand Surg Am 2014;39(3):430–5.

32. Luria S, Lenart L, Lenart B, et al. Optimal fixation of oblique scaphoid fractures: a cadaver model. J Hand Surg Am 2012;37(7):1400–4.

33. Swanstrom MM, Morse KW, Lipman JD, et al. Effect of screw perpendicularity on compression in scaphoid waist fractures. J Wrist Surg 2017;6(3):178–82.

34. Hart A, Mansuri A, Harvey EJ, et al. Central versus eccentric internal fixation of acute scaphoid fractures. J Hand Surg Am 2013;38(1):66–71.

35. Swanstrom MM, Morse KW, Lipman JD, et al. Variable bone density of scaphoid: importance of subchondral screw placement. J Wrist Surg 2018;7(1):66–70.

36. Dias JJ, Taylor M, Thompson J, et al. Radiographic signs of union of scaphoid fractures. An analysis of inter-observer agreement and reproducibility. J Bone Joint Surg Br 1988;70(2):299–301.

37. Grewal R, Suh N, Macdermid JC. Use of computed tomography to predict union and time to union in acute scaphoid fractures treated nonoperatively. J Hand Surg Am 2013;38(5):872–7.

38. Geoghegan JM, Woodruff MJ, Bhatia R, et al. Undisplaced scaphoid waist fractures: is 4 weeks' immobilisation in a below-elbow cast sufficient if a week 4 CT scan suggests fracture union? J Hand Surg Eur Vol 2009;34(5):631–7.

39. Clementson M, Jørgsholm P, Besjakov J, et al. Union of scaphoid waist fractures assessed by CT scan. J Wrist Surg 2015;4(1):49–55.

40. Grewal R, Lutz K, MacDermid JC, et al. Proximal pole scaphoid fractures: a computed tomographic assessment of outcomes. J Hand Surg Am 2016;41(1):54–8.

41. Coppage J, Hearns KA, Carlson MG. Early detection of healing of scaphoid fracture nonunions using computed tomography. Oral presentation at: American Society for Surgery of the Hand, 71st Annual Meeting. Austin, TX, September 29 - October 1, 2016.

42. Anderson LC, Gerrard DF. Ethical issues concerning New Zealand sports doctors. J Med Ethics 2005;31(2):88–92.

43. Coppage JM, Carlson MG. Expediting professional athletes' return to competition. Hand Clin 2017;33(1):9–18.

44. Husband JB. Return to play after scaphoid fractures in hockey players. Hand Clin 2012;28(3):285.

45. Carlson MG. Commentary on scaphoid fractures in basketball. Hand Clin 2012;28(3):281–2.

46. Gaston RG. Scaphoid fractures in professional football players. Hand Clin 2012;28(3):283–4.

47. Dy CJ, Khmelnitskaya E, Hearns KA, et al. Opinions regarding the management of hand and wrist injuries in elite athletes. Orthopedics 2013;36(6): 815–9.

48. Dunn WR, George MS, Churchill L, et al. Ethics in sports medicine. Am J Sports Med 2007;35(5): 840–4.

49. Johnson R. The unique ethics of sports medicine. Clin Sports Med 2004;23(2):175–82.

50. Waddington I, Roderick M. Management of medical confidentiality in English professional football clubs: some ethical problems and issues. Br J Sports Med 2002;36(2):118–23 [discussion: 123].

51. Testoni D, Hornik CP, Smith PB, et al. Sports medicine and ethics. Am J Bioeth 2013;13(10):4–12.

52. Magee JT, Almekinders LC, Taft TN. HIPAA and the team physician. Sports Medicine Update 2003;4(7): 4–8.

The Management of the Healed Scaphoid Malunion
What to Do?

Chelsea C. Boe, MD[a],*, Peter C. Amadio, MD[b],
Sanjeev Kakar, MD[b]

KEYWORDS

- Scaphoid malunion • Corrective osteotomy • DISI • Carpal collapse

KEY POINTS

- Scaphoid union alone should not be the sole goal of scaphoid fracture management and malunions, both symptomatic and asymptomatic, can occur.
- Understanding the multiplanar deformity is critical to assessing treatment options and planning surgical correction.
- Cheilectomy is a simple procedure that can help improve symptoms of dorsal impaction.
- Restoration of scaphoid anatomy by corrective osteotomy provides the best opportunity to restore more normal kinematics but comes with risk of longer recovery.
- The long-term beneficial role of surgery in the treatment of asymptomatic malunions awaits further natural history studies.

INTRODUCTION

Scaphoid malunion is rare but can result in the clinical symptoms of pain and stiffness. The altered anatomy of a malunited scaphoid can change the kinematics of the wrist and alter force transmission, resulting in the potential for increased propensity to early degenerative changes.[1–3]

A classic biomechanical study on scaphoid morphology and its effect on wrist motion demonstrated that as little as 5° of flexion through an induced fracture at the scaphoid waist results in loss of 24° of extension. At 15° of flexion deformity within the scaphoid, all radiocarpal extension is lost. With 30° of flexion deformity, all midcarpal extension is lost. It is worth noting that scaphoid deformity in this study was not radiographically measured but rather directly measured as the angle between Kirschner wires demarcating the proximal and distal fragments. The deformity induced was in a single plane and overall the study was limited by the inherent limitations of a cadaveric study, particularly in the evaluation of a dynamic entity, such as the carpus. Although an important contribution to the understanding of scaphoid malunion and resultant changes in carpal kinematics, it is difficult to translate these results directly to in vivo outcomes or quantify the degree of disability conferred.[4]

EVALUATION OF DEFORMITY

The first step in evaluation of scaphoid malunion is identification of the multidimensional nature of the deformity. Classically described is the so-called humpback deformity following scaphoid waist fracture, which results in shortening, flexion in the sagittal plane, and ulnar deviation with associated pronation of the distal fragment.[5] This tends

Disclosure Statement: The authors have no relevant conflicts of interest to disclose.
a Department of Orthopedic Surgery, Mayo Clinic, 200 1st Street Southwest, Rochester, MN 55905, USA;
b College of Medicine, Mayo Clinic, 200 1st Street Southwest, Rochester, MN 55905, USA
* Corresponding author.
E-mail address: Boe.Chelsea@mayo.edu

to occur because of the flexion moment of the distal fragment through its articulation with trapezium; the distal fragment pivots around the radio-scaphocapitate ligament while the proximal fragment is pulled into extension via an intact scapholunate ligamentous complex.[6] However, the specific degree of shortening and angulation between the proximal and distal fragments is variable, related to the location of the fracture and strength of the deforming forces as the fracture unites.

Despite numerous attempts to uniformly define radiographic measurements of scaphoid deformity, there remains no consistent standard in the literature or in practice. To review every described measurement is beyond the scope of this article, so this review focuses on measurements of historical relevance that aid in interpreting the body of literature on the topic and the most clinically relevant measures in current practice.

Modern imaging techniques, specifically computed tomography (CT) with specific scanning in the plane of the scaphoid, have improved the ability to understand scaphoid anatomy. All techniques remain prone to some error because of the complex three-dimensional bony shape that is difficult to translate into two-dimensional representations where small variations in the angle of the scanning beam can alter the reviewer's interpretation of length, height, and angulation between articular facets. This is appreciably more difficult in the setting of altered anatomy because of fracture and malunion, where defining the

central plane of the scaphoid is a challenge and leaves room for error in collection and interpretation.[7]

One of the earliest attempts to define scaphoid malunion was description of the intrascaphoid angle described by Smith and colleagues.[8] They reviewed 10 normal scaphoids to assess the normal range of angles between the proximal and distal articular surfaces in the coronal and sagittal plane, assessed by relationship of either the cortices or articular surfaces (**Fig. 1**). This angulation reflects the relative flexion of the distal pole in the sagittal plane, specifically quantifying the humpback shape of the classic waist fracture. Based on their review, abnormal was defined as greater than 42° on the lateral projection, and less than 32° or greater than 46° on the posterior-anterior projection (**Fig. 2**). The authors noted that measuring the intrascaphoid angle between the cortices, as opposed to the articular surfaces, was the most replicable and consistent in this study.[8] This group additionally reviewed a group of 46 scaphoid fractures that went on to union and applied the previous criteria to determine malunion. They found that 26 of the 46 patients had malunion defined as a lateral intrascaphoid angle (LISA) of greater than 35° and that LISA greater than 45° was predictive of fair or poor results.[1] Of note, the angles were described based on trispiral wrist tomograms and later modified to the "most central CT slice" reflecting advances in imaging technology.[9–11] The interobserver reliability of this method has

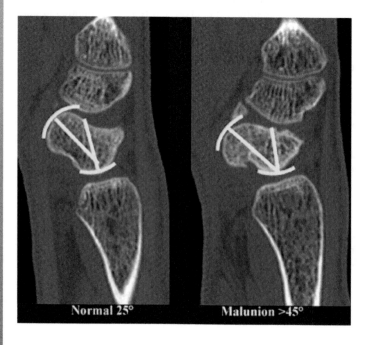

Normal 25°   Malunion >45°

Fig. 1. Lateral intrascaphoid angle by articular method, comparing normal (*left*) with abnormal (*right*). (*From* Gillette BP, Amadio PC, Kakar S. Long-term outcomes of scaphoid malunion. Hand (N Y) 2017;12(1):27; with permission.)

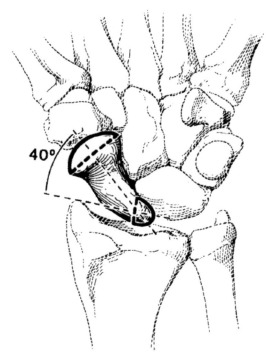

proven to be poor, with commonly reported difficulty assessing the precise end of the articular surface, despite the improved resolution with CT.[9,12,13]

The dorsal scaphoid angle is a conceptually similar evaluation, with the angle measured between lines formed along the dorsal cortex of the scaphoid, tangential to the flattest portion of the proximal and distal halves.[9] Unfortunately, given the curved nature of the dorsal cortex of the scaphoid and subjective interpretation of the flattest portion of cortex and similar variability dependent on the specific slice selected on CT, interobserver reliability for this measure remains poor.[7,9]

To describe shortening and angulation of the scaphoid, the calculated height-to-length ratio (HLR) has been used, based on the most central slice through the scaphoid on CT scan. To measure the height-to-length ratio, a line is drawn along the volar scaphoid and maximal length is measured along this line. A perpendicular line is drawn on the same CT slice and maximal height measured.[9] Although not a specific measure of angulation between the articular facets, it can signify deformity of the scaphoid and predict the potential for dorsal intercalated segment instability (DISI) when the ratio exceeds 0.73.[14] This measure seems to have the best interobserver reliability relative to the LISA and dorsal cortical angle because of the limited observer interpretation.[9,11] There remains some intraobserver variability, likely attributable to the decision on which specific slice represents the most central through the axis of the scaphoid.[7,9] The interobserver and intraobserver variability is substantially increased when "most central slice" is agreed on.[12] This measure can also be applied in the coronal plane, elucidating deformity hidden by measures in a single plane.[15]

The most recent advances in scaphoid imaging relate to three-dimensional modeling and reconstructions. The ability to recreate the unique and variable shape of the scaphoid independent of scanning angle allows the most comprehensive imaging. In addition, physical models are produced for evaluation and ultimately, surgical planning (**Fig. 3**). These models reduce reliance on indirect measures of deformity, such as fluoroscopy, which are best regarded as poor in evaluation of rotational deformity.[16] Previous evaluations of normal scaphoids have shown that there is a high correlation (correlation coefficient >0.92) between contralateral scaphoids in regard to volume, surface area, and length, thus validating the use of a mirrored template. Of note, there is a higher degree of variability in men, and scaphoid length can differ by 1.9 mm comparing left and right.[17] The biomechanical and clinical significance of this difference is

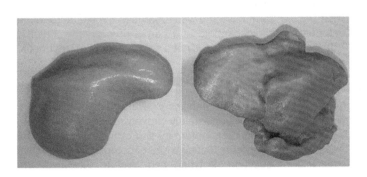

Fig. 3. Three-dimensional models of normal and malunited contralateral scaphoid.

certainly not well understood, limiting the ability to comment on how these data should be interpreted. There may be a future role for computer-generated quantification of metrics, such as maximal height and length, which would not be subject to the error of defining and assessing a single two-dimensional representation.

Regardless of the method used to evaluate scaphoid deformity, the measurements tend to be unreliable leading some authors to deduce that conclusions drawn from these data would have to be regarded as speculative.[7] Certainly, increased attention to these measures has perhaps elucidated previously unrecognized deformity in healed scaphoid fractures and begs the question of clinical relevance.

DOES MALUNION MATTER?

Despite the documented implications on carpal motion with even limited degrees of angular deformity, several studies have demonstrated that not all malunions are symptomatic.[12,18,19] Information about the natural history of malunion is gleaned from the literature on scaphoid nonunion. An investigation of 25 patients with 11 years average follow-up after Russe bone grafting for management of nonunion revealed no difference in subjective outcome regardless of persistent deformity, defined as LISA greater than 45° on CT scan of the scaphoid at most recent follow-up.[2] Overall 81% of these healed fractures were considered malunited by this measure. This malunited population did have highly significant decrease in grip strength and arc of motion, which correlated with the degree of deformity although not with subjective outcomes.[2] A similar group of 25 patients following treatment of scaphoid nonunion with follow-up of 81 months were evaluated for malunion using the more reliable and reproducible HLR. The authors found that 15 of the 25 patients were malunited. However, they demonstrated no difference in outcome, namely range of motion, grip strength, and Disabilities of the Arm, Shoulder and Hand or Mayo Wrist Scores, regardless of deformity.[20] It is worth noting that in this study, deformity was defined as HLR greater than 0.6, which is a lower threshold for defining deformity than typically associated with DISI.[14] It was concluded that the morphology of the scaphoid had no apparent impact on the outcome of scaphoid fracture in the clinical setting. Perhaps this study identifies a group of radiographically identifiable malunion that remains clinically silent, further substantiating that our metrics for determining malunion are either insufficient measures or fail to capture the relevant altered mechanical properties of the scaphoid that generate clinical symptoms.

In one of the larger case series on long term outcomes specifically focusing on scaphoid malunion, 17 patients with a diagnosis of scaphoid malunion and follow-up of greater than 10 years were retrospectively evaluated. The authors found no difference in Quick Disabilities of the Arm, Shoulder and Hand or Patient Rated Wrist Evaluation scores between patients treated with corrective osteotomy, salvage procedures (dorsal cheilectomy, radial styloidectomy or scaphoidectomy, and four-corner fusion), and nonoperative management.[6] However, in the nonoperative group, 50% of patients had poor outcome and 50% had an excellent outcome at 21.4 years average follow-up.[6] This suggests that although not all malunions are symptomatic, it is a mistake to conclude that all malunions are asymptomatic. This underscores the need to better understand what patient factors, coexisting conditions, or mechanical properties of the malunion result in clinical symptoms.

Although there is evidence to suggest that malunion alone does not correlate with symptoms, the obviously altered carpal kinematics seems to predispose the wrist to degenerative changes.[1–3] DISI and carpal collapse are part of the natural history of scaphoid dysfunction. Previous authors have demonstrated a highly significant linear relationship between deformity of the scaphoid and carpal collapse[2] and restriction of motion and decreased grip strength.[3] A case series of 46 patients with average follow-up of 44.7 months postunion revealed that patients with LISA exceeding 45° achieved what was graded as a satisfactory clinical outcome in only 27% of cases. Of those in the group with the increased LISA, 54% developed post-traumatic degenerative joint disease. This is compared with 83% of patients achieving a satisfactory clinical outcome and only 22% with evidence of posttraumatic degenerative joint disease in the group with LISA less than 45°.[1] This would seem to clearly suggest that there are ramifications of a scaphoid healed in a malunited position, in overall clinical outcome and projected long-term outcome with regards to the character of the radioscaphoid and carpal articulations. Fracture healing alone is not a sufficient goal of treatment.

TREATMENT OF MALUNION

The inconsistencies in evaluation, definition, and lack of consistently proven relationship between measurable deformity and clinical symptoms and long-term sequelae further complicate the surgical question of when and how to intervene. The spectrum of described surgical treatment ranges from corrective osteotomy to salvage procedures, such as dorsal cheilectomy, radial styloidectomy, neurectomy, or scaphoidectomy and four-corner fusion.

In the series published by Gilette and colleagues,[6] five patients were treated with dorsal cheilectomy and/or radial styloidectomy, although the results of that procedure are not directly compared with alternate salvage procedures or corrective osteotomy limiting direct conclusions. At the time of this review, neither evaluation of biomechanical alterations following cheilectomy nor comparison studies between dorsal cheilectomy and osteotomy and correction of malunion were available for review. It is unclear how dorsal cheilectomy or radial styloidectomy would significantly alter the underlying kinematics of the carpus, although removal of the dorsal prominence may provide some relief from impingement or soft tissue irritation.

Several authors have reported techniques and small case series evaluating the outcomes of scaphoid osteotomy and bone grafting for correction of malunion.[3,21-24] Given that the most common deformity is a flexion or "humpback" deformity, this often involves wedge grafting to the volar aspect of the scaphoid. An osteotomy is created at the previous fracture site, or apex of deformity (**Fig. 4**), and the scaphoid malunion is corrected indirectly by correcting the DISI deformity, as described by Lynch and Linscheid.[23] Following scaphoid osteotomy, the wrist is palmar flexed and ulnarly deviated to reduce the DISI as evaluated by the relative extension of the lunate. A 0.062-inch Kirschner wire is passed from the radial metaphysis to the neutrally aligned lunate to maintain the reduction. A structural, wedge-shaped graft, often harvested from the iliac crest, is shaped to fill the defect and transfixed with a cannulated screw or Kirschner wires.[25,26] Alternate grafts include radial metaphyseal cortical cancellous graft[27] or a structural, vascularized graft, such as the medial femoral condyle.[28] In the series of five patients reported by Lynch and Linscheid,[23] average grip strength doubled from 16 kg to 32 kg, Mayo wrist score improved by 56 points, and total arc of motion improved by 29° at nearly 9 years of follow-up.[23]

Fernandez and colleagues[22] evaluated three patients at a minimum of 4 years of follow-up after corrective scaphoid osteotomy and noted that all patients had improvement in motion and grip strength, were pain-free, and were satisfied with the procedure. All had returned in an unlimited capacity to their preoperative occupation. In a series of 13 patients treated with similar corrective

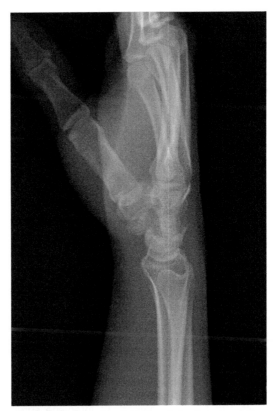

Fig. 4. A 22-year-old, right hand–dominant male patient with significant DISI deformity following scaphoid fracture and subsequent malunion.

osteotomy, motion and grip were improved to approximately 80% of the contralateral side and 85% were rated as good or excellent by Mayo Wrist Score at 42 months follow-up.[21] Another series of seven patients demonstrated improvement of arc of motion and grip strength to 85% or better compared with the contralateral side and effectively corrected the radiolunate angle to within 10° of the contralateral side at nearly 30 months follow-up.[3] Correction of carpal alignment in the form of radiolunate and scapholunate was also significant in a series of 24 patients, with an average Mayo Wrist Score of 81.2 at 19.4 months follow-up.[24] Iatrogenic avascular necrosis has not manifested in the reported literature.[3,22-24,29] There has been a recent trend in the use of anatomic scaphoid plates to correct these deformities because it is technically difficult to know how much correction is needed and prevent overstuffing of the joint, although data detailing or comparing results to cannulated screw fixation are lacking.

Future investigation is focused on using three-dimensional technology and modeling capabilities to advance detailed evaluation of deformity. This technology has applications inside the operating room in the form of customized surgical guides. These guides allow for precise planning and correction in multiple planes that is not dependent on crude, two-dimensional images and subjective assessments of alignment available intraoperatively.[30,31] Scaphoid osteotomy and reconstruction is based on indirect measures of deformity correction and three-dimensional printing and custom cutting guide applications allow for highly exacting manipulation and correction of the morphology to mimic the contralateral side. This represents an opportunity to achieve the goal of scaphoid fracture care that is not merely union, but restoration of normal anatomy and presumably kinematics.

SUMMARY

Historically, the priority in the treatment of scaphoid fractures has been obtaining bony union. However, increased recognition of the ramifications of altered scaphoid anatomy following malunion have challenged the dogma that healing alone is sufficient. Scaphoid malunion can lead to pain and stiffness. Not all malunions are symptomatic and, based on the long-term data, some of these remain asymptomatic. To intervene surgically requires an understanding of the deformity; the technical ability to make an appropriate correction; and willingness for surgeon and patient to accept the possible complications, which may require progression to salvage operations. This emphasizes the importance of the art of medicine, an understanding of the patient's motivations and expectations, and a frank discussion of the risks and potential benefits of such an intervention.

In an asymptomatic patient, there is no clear consensus regarding the appropriate treatment and thus it is difficult to advocate for the risk and recovery associated with an osteotomy and correction.[2,32] Certainly there are specific cases where this would be considered and should be presented to the patient for shared decision making. One would deduce that there is an advantage of restoring normal anatomy and preventing carpal collapse and progression of degenerative joint disease, although the clinical evidence does not support that all patients progress in this manner.[21,33] Clearly, there is a need to better understand those patients for whom early intervention may postpone salvage procedures or obviate them entirely.

In a symptomatic patient, limited interventions, such as cheilectomy, could be considered and discussed, although with appropriately tempered expectations. If the patient is interested in motion

preservation and advanced degenerative changes are absent, then there is clearly a role for osteotomy with structural bone graft to restore anatomy. The outcomes are promising in regards to healing of the osteotomy, and demonstrable improvements in pain, motion, and strength. Substantially improved functional scores are consistently obtained with scaphoid reconstruction. Given the relative equipoise in the treatment plan, there is a critical need for individualized treatment dependent on the wishes, needs, and demands of each patient.

REFERENCES

1. Amadio PC, Berquist TH, Smith DK, et al. Scaphoid malunion. J Hand Surg Am 1989;14(4):679–87.
2. Jiranek WA, Ruby LK, Millender LB, et al. Long-term results after Russe bone-grafting: the effect of malunion of the scaphoid. J Bone Joint Surg Am 1992; 74(8):1217–28.
3. Nakamura P, Imaeda T, Miura T. Scaphoid malunion. J Bone Joint Surg Br 1991;73(1):134–7.
4. Burgess RC. The effect of a simulated scaphoid malunion on wrist motion. J Hand Surg Am 1987; 12(5 Pt 1):774–6.
5. Barton NJ. Twenty questions about scaphoid fractures. J Hand Surg Br 1992;17(3):289–310.
6. Gillette BP, Amadio PC, Kakar S. Long-term outcomes of scaphoid malunion. Hand (N Y) 2017; 12(1):26–30.
7. Ring D, Patterson JD, Levitz S, et al. Both scanning plane and observer affect measurements of scaphoid deformity. J Hand Surg Am 2005;30(4): 696–701.
8. Smith DK, Linscheid RL, Amadio PC, et al. Scaphoid anatomy: evaluation with complex motion tomography. Radiology 1989;173(1):177–80.
9. Bain GI, Bennett JD, MacDermid JC, et al. Measurement of the scaphoid humpback deformity using longitudinal computed tomography: intra- and interobserver variability using various measurement techniques. J Hand Surg Am 1998;23(1): 76–81.
10. Bain GI, Bennett JD, Richards RS, et al. Longitudinal computed tomography of the scaphoid: a new technique. Skeletal Radiol 1995;24(4):271–3.
11. Garcia-Elias M, An KN, Amadio PC, et al. Reliability of carpal angle determinations. J Hand Surg Am 1989;14(6):1017–21.
12. Forward DP, Singh HP, Dawson S, et al. The clinical outcome of scaphoid fracture malunion at 1 year. J Hand Surg Eur Vol 2009;34(1):40–6.
13. Lozano-Calderon S, Blazar P, Zurakowski D, et al. Diagnosis of scaphoid fracture displacement with radiography and computed tomography. J Bone Joint Surg Am 2006;88(12):2695–703.

14. Kim JH, Lee KH, Lee BG, et al. Dorsal intercalated segmental instability associated with malunion of a reconstructed scaphoid. J Hand Surg Eur Vol 2017;42(3):240–5.

15. Ten Berg PW, Dobbe JG, Horbach SE, et al. Analysis of deformity in scaphoid non-unions using two- and three-dimensional imaging. J Hand Surg Eur Vol 2016;41(7):719–26.

16. Haefeli M, Schaefer DJ, Schumacher R, et al. Titanium template for scaphoid reconstruction. J Hand Surg Eur Vol 2015;40(5):526–33.

17. Letta C, Schweizer A, Furnstahl P. Quantification of contralateral differences of the scaphoid: a comparison of bone geometry in three dimensions. Anat Res Int 2014;2014:904275.

18. Megerle K, Harenberg PS, Germann G, et al. Scaphoid morphology and clinical outcomes in scaphoid reconstructions. Injury 2012;43(3):306–10.

19. Roh YH, Noh JH, Lee BK, et al. Reliability and validity of carpal alignment measurements in evaluating deformities of scaphoid fractures. Arch Orthop Trauma Surg 2014;134(6):887–93.

20. Lee CH, Lee KH, Lee BG, et al. Clinical outcome of scaphoid malunion as a result of scaphoid fracture nonunion surgical treatment: a 5-year minimum follow-up study. Orthop Traumatol Surg Res 2015; 101(3):359–63.

21. El-Karef EA. Corrective osteotomy for symptomatic scaphoid malunion. Injury 2005;36(12):1440–8.

22. Fernandez DL, Martin CJ, Gonzalez del Pino J. Scaphoid malunion. The significance of rotational malalignment. J Hand Surg Br 1998;23(6):771–5.

23. Lynch NM, Linscheid RL. Corrective osteotomy for scaphoid malunion: technique and long-term follow-up evaluation. J Hand Surg Am 1997;22(1): 35–43.

24. Tsuyuguchi Y, Murase T, Hidaka N, et al. Anterior wedge-shaped bone graft for old scaphoid fractures or non-unions. An analysis of relevant carpal alignment. J Hand Surg Br 1995;20(2):194–200.

25. Fisk GR. Carpal instability and the fractured scaphoid. Ann R Coll Surg Engl 1970;46(2):63–76.

26. Fisk GR. An overview of injuries of the wrist. Clin Orthop Relat Res 1980;(149):137–44.

27. Aguilella L, Garcia-Elias M. The anterolateral corner of the radial metaphysis as a source of bone graft for the treatment of scaphoid nonunion. J Hand Surg Am 2012;37(6):1258–62.

28. Jones DB Jr, Burger H, Bishop AT, et al. Treatment of scaphoid waist nonunions with an avascular proximal pole and carpal collapse. A comparison of two vascularized bone grafts. J Bone Joint Surg Am 2008;90(12):2616–25.

29. Birchard D, Pichora D. Experimental corrective scaphoid osteotomy for scaphoid malunion with abnormal wrist mechanics. J Hand Surg Am 1990; 15(6):863–8.

30. Schweizer A, Furnstahl P, Nagy L. Three-dimensional computed tomographic analysis of 11 scaphoid waist nonunions. J Hand Surg Am 2012; 37(6):1151–8.

31. Schweizer A, Furnstahl P, Nagy L. Three-dimensional correction of distal radius intra-articular malunions using patient-specific drill guides. J Hand Surg Am 2013;38(12):2339–47.

32. Nakamura R. Scaphoid mal-union: current concept and perspectives. Hand Surg 2000;5(2):155–60.

33. Mathoulin CL, Arianni M. Treatment of the scaphoid humpback deformity: is correction of the dorsal intercalated segment instability deformity critical? J Hand Surg Eur Vol 2018;43(1):13–23.

Moving?

Make sure your subscription moves with you!

To notify us of your new address, find your **Clinics Account Number** (located on your mailing label above your name), and contact customer service at:

Email: journalscustomerservice-usa@elsevier.com

800-654-2452 (subscribers in the U.S. & Canada)
314-447-8871 (subscribers outside of the U.S. & Canada)

Fax number: 314-447-8029

Elsevier Health Sciences Division
Subscription Customer Service
3251 Riverport Lane
Maryland Heights, MO 63043

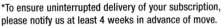

*To ensure uninterrupted delivery of your subscription, please notify us at least 4 weeks in advance of move.

ELSEVIER

Printed and bound by CPI Group (UK) Ltd, Croydon, CR0 4YY

03/10/2024

01040370-0014